Specialized Strength Training

Winning Workouts
for Specific Populations

Wayne L. Westcott, Ph.D.

Susan F. Ramsden

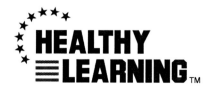

Library of Congress Cataloging-in-Publication Data

Westcott, Wayne L., 1949-
    Specialized strength training: winning workouts for specific
populations / Wayne Westcott, Susan Ramsden, and Nautilus
International.
        p.   cm.
    Includes bibliographical references.
    ISBN: 1-58518-408-X
        1. Physical fitness. 2. Exercise. 3. Nautilus weight training.
    I. Nautilus International (Firm) II. Title.

Library of Congress Catalog Card Number: 00-111337

                                                                    CIP

ISBN: 1-58518-408-X

Copyright © 2001 by Nautilus International, Inc.

Interior design and layout by Kim Maxey.
Cover design by Studio J Art & Design.

Printed in the United States of America.

Healthy Learning
P.O. Box 1828
Monterey, CA 93942
Tel: (831) 372-6077
Fax: (831) 372-6075
www.healthylearning.com

Contents

Acknowledgments

It is our privilege to acknowledge the following individuals for their invaluable assistance in producing this manuscript. We first want to thank Dr. Rick Frey, Dr. Jim Peterson, and Kim McFarland Maxey, our talented and patient editors, for their professional expertise and personal encouragement throughout the publishing process. We are indebted to Rita LaRosa Loud, our associate research director, for her outstanding leadership with our class instructors and program participants. We also thank Debra Wein, M.S., R.D. and Karen Leary for helping Rita develop the nutrition education component of our weight loss program. Special appreciation is given to Claudia Westcott, Gayle Laring, Tracy D'Arpino, and their instructional staff for managing a model Nautilus Fitness Center. We are also grateful to our executive directors at the South Shore YMCA, Ralph Yohe, Mary Hurley, and Bill Johnson, for their continuing support of our studies, programs and projects. We credit the creation of this book to Jim Teatum, president of Nautilus, and his fine associates, for encouraging and enabling our efforts in practical research, training design and program development. We express our sincere appreciation to the thousands of individuals who have wholeheartedly participated in our research programs over the past 15 years, teaching us the important training information that we share in this text. Finally, we thank God for the privilege of writing a book on specialized strength training, and we hope you find it a useful resource in your fitness facility.

Introduction

As we enter the 21st Century, we are pleased with the progress that has been made in the field of strength training. Research studies have supported the training principles associated with sensible strength exercise. These include relatively infrequent workouts (two or three sessions per week), relatively brief workouts (one set of 8 to 12 repetitions for 8 to 12 exercises), relatively slow movement speed (six or more seconds per repetition), relatively full movement range (through extended and flexed joint positions), and relatively small progressions (1 to 3-pound weightload increases).

We are also encouraged by the higher levels of knowledge, teaching skills and enthusiasm exhibited by exercise instructors and personal trainers, as well as by the advancements in the fitness profession. There has never been a better time for youth, adults, seniors, and people with disabilities to begin an effective exercise program with competent supervision, excellent equipment, and sound training guidelines.

However, motivating individuals who are not presently strength training to initiate a personal exercise program is frequently a futile experience. Many people are simply too intimidated to venture into even the finest fitness facility because they feel too old, too young, too heavy, too light, too uncoordinated or too unclear about proper training procedures, appropriate exercise attire, and related issues. While this is most unfortunate, it is a fact that we must address in a persuasive and productive manner. Towards this end, we have directed most of our research efforts over the past 15 years to reaching and teaching previously sedentary individuals with respect to strength training. While we have encountered a few frustrations, the majority of our studies have been successful, and we have learned a great deal about attaining and maintaining new strength training participants.

Our studies have focused on sedentary adults, seniors, youth, golfers, time-pressured people, overweight individuals, and advanced trainees. We have also worked extensively with cardiac rehabilitation patients and people with various disabilities. In addition, we have conducted cutting-edge research on several factors that appear to enhance strength development and overall physical fitness, such as the integration of strength and endurance training and the interaction of strength and stretching exercise.

These studies, many of which have been conducted over several years with hundreds of participants, are the foundation for our research-based training recommendations and program implementation strategies. While we have acquired a wealth of information about safe, effective and efficient strength training, we have learned even more about attracting non-exercisers into targeted fitness programs.

For example, we have proven over and over the superiority of a separate exercise facility, small classes with close supervision, and simple training protocols for beginning exercisers. By so doing, we encourage people to participate without fear or embarrassment, and help them develop the competence and confidence necessary to enjoy their exercise experiences. The results have been highly reinforcing, with positive attitudes and consistent attendance from almost all of our program participants.

Basically, everyone has the same major muscle groups and therefore benefits from a basic strength training program that effectively addresses all of these muscles in a balanced manner. However, upon attaining a reasonable level of comprehensive muscular conditioning it is typically advantageous to train with a more specialized approach. The basic intent of this book is to present practical and well-researched strength training programs that serve specific purposes and populations. Perhaps most important, you will find the recommended programs are easy to implement in essentially any well-equipped and well-staffed fitness facility.

The information is presented in the following order and includes a variety of strength training programs for people with different characteristics and fitness objectives. Chapter One addresses the largest segment of the population, namely sedentary adults who make up between 70 and 90 percent of the men and women in our automated society. In this chapter we present the basic approach to sensible strength exercise that has worked so well for thousands of our research participants over the past 15 years.

The second chapter reduces the standard training protocol to its minimum requirements providing a more time-efficient approach to strength development. Fortunately, these brief workouts have proven highly effective for the time-pressured people who regularly incorporate them into their busy lifestyles.

Chapter Three presents the only permanent solution to the pervasive problem of obesity. While some diets may provide temporary reductions in bodyweight, they do not address the muscle loss that is largely responsible for the fat gain. To restore desirable body composition and metabolic rate, strength training is an absolutely essential component of the reshaping program. Our Nautilus Weight Loss Program recently received the NOVA 7 Award for Program Excellence from *Fitness Management Magazine,* underscoring the importance of strength training for attaining and maintaining ideal bodyweight.

The fourth chapter is directed towards men and women between the ages of 50 and 100. In this section we present the key concepts and components of functional strength training for older adults. The exercise guidelines are derived from several years of research with senior subjects, and have an excellent record with respect to providing safe and successful strength training experiences. In fact, more than 90 percent of the senior program participants continued to strength train after completing just 10 weeks of classes in our exercise center.

Chapter Five addresses the other end of the age continuum, namely youth strength training. We have studied strength training in children since 1985, and have gained a greater understanding of effective exercise guidelines for boys and girls. For example, we have learned that preadolescents respond better to training protocols using more repetitions with moderate weightloads than to programs using fewer repetitions with heavy weightloads. In this chapter we present important information on safe, practical and productive strength training programs for youth that have proven effective and enjoyable for both active and sedentary boys and girls.

Chapter Six is directed towards a specific sport that is played by more than 25 million men and women of all ages. Golf is a great game, but it provides very little fitness benefit and poses a high risk of injury due to the explosive action of the golf swing. Our research has shown that a relatively brief program of strength and stretching exercise can have a profound positive effect on golfers' body composition, blood pressure, muscle strength, and driving ability (club head speed), as well as assist with injury prevention and enhance playing enjoyment.

We have devoted Chapter Seven to strength training enthusiasts who have reached a plateau with their standard exercise program. This section addresses advanced training techniques through a variety of high-intensity exercise protocols. These include slow-positive training, slow-negative training, breakdown training, assisted training, and pre-exhaustion training. Several studies have demonstrated excellent strength gains and body composition improvements resulting from just six weeks of high-intensity training.

Chapters Eight and Nine present research and recommendations for people who were previously precluded from participating in strength training activities. Chapter Eight provides detailed information on a heart-healthy strength training program for cardiac rehabilitation patients. Chapter Nine discusses appropriate upper-body strength training programs for people in wheelchairs. We explain how to perform numerous exercises on both specially-designed equipment (Bow Flex Versa Trainer) and standard Nautilus machines that have proven highly-effective for wheelchair users.

Our final chapter, titled New Discoveries and Directions, presents our most recent research that is relevant to program design and implementation. These studies include integrating strength and endurance exercise, combining strength and stretching exercise, exercise introduction based on participants' perceived exertion, and strength training frequency. The results of these studies have proven most helpful in new program development, such as the *Nautilus Expressway Training Program* that incorporates strength, flexibility and endurance exercise into a brief but comprehensive conditioning session.

As you can see, this text is written for fitness professionals who want to reach and teach various populations of non-exercisers, but who don't have time to research and develop several group-specific strength training programs. We trust that our work in these areas will be helpful for implementing participant-appropriate exercise programs with user-friendly training protocols. Of course, we do not expect each program model to be perfect for every situation, but we hope that you will need to make only minor adaptations to successfully introduce your new members to purposeful strength training.

Although our facility is equipped with Nautilus machines, the programs presented in this text may be conducted with other types of resistance apparatus, including various brands of weightstack machines, air-pressure machines, hydraulic machines, electronic machines, barbells, dumbbells, elastic tubing, and even bodyweight. Simply use the same exercise movements, training principles and program components, and your participants should attain similar results. We hope that you and your clients will find each program to be a safe, effective and efficient means for achieving its stated objectives.

Chapter 1

Sedentary Solutions

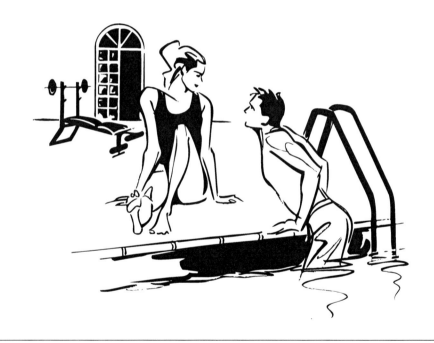

Basic Strength Program for Average Adults

When Nautilus equipment was first introduced in 1970, it was unique in many respects. The well-constructed weightstack machines featured rotary movements and direct resistance to better isolate individual muscle groups. They also provided cam and chain mechanisms to automatically vary the resistance in accordance with each muscle's strength curve, giving proportionately less resistance in weaker positions and proportionately more resistance in stronger positions.

While these design characteristics were nothing short of striking, they were actually less revolutionary than the proposed training principles for using the new Nautilus machines. According to the equipment designer, Arthur Jones, muscle strength could be best enhanced by performing just one set of each exercise. He advised training at a slow movement speed, through a full movement range, with a weightload that could be performed between 8 and 12 repetitions.

Although it was a simple and sensible exercise protocol, most strength experts were unimpressed with the Nautilus training procedures. However, almost three decades of research have revealed these basic recommendations to be safe and productive for muscle development (Westcott 1995b). Because they are both effective and efficient, several prominent national associations presently promote these strength training principles. Consider the recently-released guidelines for strength exercise from the prestigious *American College of Sports Medicine (ACSM 1998)*.

> *"Resistance training should be an integral part of an adult fitness program and of a sufficient intensity to enhance strength, muscular endurance, and maintain fat-free mass (FFM). Resistance training should be progressive in nature, individualized, and provide a stimulus to all the major muscle groups. One set of 8-10 exercises that conditions the major muscle groups 2-3 days a week is recommended. Multiple-set regimens may provide greater benefits if time allows. Most persons should complete 8-12 repetitions of each exercise; however, for older and more frail persons (approximately 50-60 years of age and above), 10-15 repetitions may be more appropriate."*

Results

What kind of results can your clients attain by following these strength training principles? Over the past several years we have conducted several research studies with adults, seniors, and children consistent with the American College of Sports Medicine exercise guidelines. In every program, the participants experienced excellent gains in muscle strength and impressive improvements in body composition. On average, our adult exercisers increased their muscle strength by more than 40 percent, added 2.4 pounds of muscle, and lost 4.4 pounds of fat over an eight-week training period (Westcott and Guy 1996). Table 1-1 details the findings from our study with 1,132 young, middle-age, and older adults.

	Body Weight (lbs.)	Percent Fat (%)	Fat Weight (lbs)	Lean Weight (lbs)	Mean Blood Pressure (mm Hg)
Men (383)	-2.7	-2.7	-6.4	+3.7	-4.5
Women (749)	-1.8	-1.8	-3.4	+1.7	-3.9
21-40 Yrs. (238)	-2.6	-2.3	-4.9	+2.3	-3.9
41-60 Yrs. (553)	-2.0	-2.1	-4.4	+2.3	-2.5
61 – 80 Yrs. (341)	-1.7	-2.0	-4.1	+2.4	-5.0
Total (1,132)	**-2.1**	**-2.1**	**-4.4**	**+2.4**	**-3.6**

Table 1-1   Results of 8-week basic exercise program including 24 minutes of strength training (12 Nautilus machines) and 20 minutes of endurance training (treadmill walking or stationary cycling) with 1132 subjects.

These results are at least as good as those attained using more demanding and complex exercise protocols, indicating that a brief strength training program can be highly effective for muscle conditioning. Perhaps just as important, participants have been pleased with both the exercise process and the training product, with over 90 percent continuing their workouts after completing the basic strength training program.

Basic Strength Training Program

Our basic strength training program is performed on Nautilus machines, and includes the 12 exercises presented in Table 1-2. You will note that we pair exercises for opposing muscles, starting with the legs and progressing to the upper body, arms, midsection, and neck groups. As we stated in the introduction, you may perform the basic exercises on other types of resistance equipment.

We do one set of each exercise, with a weightload that can be lifted between 8 and 12 repetitions. Each repetition is performed at a moderate movement speed (about 6 seconds) and through a full movement range. When 12 repetitions can be completed in proper form, the weightload is increased by a small amount (5 percent or less). The participants train either two or three days per week depending on personal preference. Our studies have shown almost 90 percent as much benefit from twice-a-week training as three-day-a-week training (see Table 1-3).

Nautilus Exercise	Major Muscle Groups
Leg Extension	Quadriceps
Leg Curl	Hamstrings
Leg Press	Quadriceps, Hamstrings, Gluteals
Chest Cross	Pectoralis Major
Super Pullover	Latissimus Dorsi
Lateral Raise	Deltoids
Biceps Curl	Biceps
Triceps Extension	Triceps
Low Back	Erector Spinae
Abdominal	Rectus Abdominis
Neck Flexion	Neck Flexors
Neck Extension	Neck Extensors

Table 1-2   Nautilus exercises included in the basic strength training program.*

You may have noticed that some major muscles, such as the calves, are not addressed in our basic strength training program. You may, of course, add the calf machine or other exercises that you consider essential to your program. Just be careful not to introduce too many exercises to beginning strength trainers.

	Body Weight (lbs.)	Percent Fat (%)	Fat Weight (lbs)	Lean Weight (lbs)	Mean Blood Pressure (mm Hg)
2 Days (416)	-1.8	-2.0	-4.0	+2.2	-5.1
3 Days (716)	-2.1	-2.2	-4.6	+2.5	-3.4

Table 1-3   Body composition changes following 8 weeks of training 2 or 3 days per week (1132 subjects).

The basic training program is relatively time-efficient, depending of course on the recovery period between exercises. Assuming about a minute to perform each exercise and about a minute between exercises, the basic Nautilus workout requires only 24 minutes for completion.

Program Development

So how do you develop a basic strength training program in your workout facility? The first step is to determine your training philosophy. The second step is to design a management system that puts your training philosophy into practice. This is typically presented in the form of a member brochure that clearly describes the exercise principles and training procedures to be used in your fitness facility. We believe our member brochure meets these criteria, and because we have had many requests to use this information we include it for your review. You are welcome to reproduce any or all of this material as you create a management philosophy brochure for members of your exercise facility.

How We Manage Our Nautilus Fitness Facility

The South Shore YMCA is pleased to provide a large and well-managed Nautilus Fitness Center. We feature four full lines of the newest Nautilus strength training machines and highly qualified instructors during all hours of operation.

Our goal is for every participant to experience a safe, effective and efficient exercise session during every visit to our facility. We want your workout to have a minimum amount of waiting time and a maximum amount of activity time. To best ensure this type of exercise environment we provide a structured training facility and strict training procedures.

Structured Training Facility

As you enter our fitness facility you will see several lines of 12 to 14 Nautilus machines, arranged in order of larger to smaller muscles groups. Our training policy is to use the machines in this order, beginning with the muscles of the legs and progressing to the muscles of the upper body, arms, midsection, and neck.

Our facility training protocol is to perform one set of each exercise, then to spray and dry the machine upholstery after use. Under certain circumstances it is permissible to skip a particular machine, but you must not cut-off another exerciser when entering the Nautilus line. Always move at least two machines ahead of the next exerciser to facilitate training flow.

Our structured approach to exercise includes careful records of all training activities. Please write down your training weightloads and repetitions for each Nautilus exercise on your personal workout card.

(continued)

Strict Training Procedures

We have conducted several studies on strength training, including the optimum exercise frequency, exercise sets, exercise repetitions, exercise speed, and exercise order. Our research results are consistent with the strength training recommendations of the American College of Sports Medicine (ACSM 1998), the American Council on Exercise (Sudy 1991), the YMCA of the USA (Westcott 1987), and the Nautilus Corporation (Westcott and Urmston 1995). These are essentially as follows:

1. Perform one exercise for each major muscle group in order from larger to smaller.
2. Perform one set of each exercise.
3. Use a weightload that you can lift between 8 and 12 repetitions in good form.
4. Increase the weightload by 5 percent or less when you can complete 12 repetitions.
5. Perform every repetition through a full range of pain-free joint movement.
6. Perform every repetition in a controlled manner, typically 2 seconds for each lifting action and 4 seconds for each lowering action.
7. Exhale during each lifting movement and inhale during each lowering movement.
8. Train two or three nonconsecutive days per week.

Because even the most carefully controlled strength workout carries a small risk of injury, we require every participant to complete our medical history form before training in the Nautilus Fitness Facility. If any exercise contraindications are evident, we request clearance from your personal physician.

Qualified Instructional Staff

To help you train properly and productively, we provide continuous staffing in the Nautilus Fitness Facility. Our staff are highly qualified, and serve two important functions. Their first responsibility is competent exercise instruction, and their second responsibility is attentive exercise supervision.

Please cooperate with our Nautilus instructors, accept their training advice, and ask them questions. Just remember that they are not qualified to give you medical recommendations. Our Nautilus staff are here to serve you, and their highest priority is to ensure a safe, effective, and efficient exercise experience for every participant.

Daily Equipment Maintenance

Because we want our exercise equipment to function at the showroom level, we perform daily maintenance procedures on all of the Nautilus machines. In addition, every Nautilus machine is thoroughly overhauled four times a year. Our main maintenance objective is to stop trouble before it starts. However, if you notice any equipment-related problems, please notify a Nautilus instructor immediately.

Member Orientation

To best prepare you for safe and successful strength training experiences, we require each member to participate in an orientation session before starting your exercise program. The 40-minute orientation sessions are offered every weekday at 12:00 noon and 6:00 p.m. Each orientation session includes an informative slide presentation on training principles and procedures, as well as administration of the medical history form, All About Exercise booklet, and personal workout card. This is followed by a question-answer opportunity to make sure everyone understands our training philosophy.

Immediately after the orientation session, you sign-up for your first one-on-one training session with a Nautilus instructor. You may schedule as many training sessions as necessary to develop competence and confidence in your personal exercise program.

An optional but highly recommended component of the orientation program is the personal fitness assessment. This includes measures of body composition, blood pressure, muscular strength, cardiovascular endurance, and joint flexibility.

Member Education

Beginning with the orientation session, we do our best to offer you relevant exercise information. You will receive our training manual All About Exercise that should serve as a practical workout resource. You may request any of Dr. Westcott's article reprints (over 400 available), or purchase any of Dr. Westcott's fitness books at cost. The Keeping Fit bulletin board displays Dr. Westcott's current newspaper column and recently published fitness articles.

In addition, our Nautilus instructors are knowledgeable in the area of exercise and fitness. Please feel free to discuss your training program or related matters with them at any time.

Member Motivation

Because we believe that proper exercise enhances the quality and quantity of your life, we want you to exercise on a regular basis. We are interested in both your training process and your training product. That is, we want you to have enjoyable exercise experiences and excellent exercise results.

We hope that you are pleased with our spacious fitness facilities and state-of-the-art exercise equipment. We also hope that you find our training atmosphere pleasant and our instructor attitudes positive. *(continued)*

Whether you are a beginner, intermediate, or advanced exerciser, our purpose is to help you achieve your fitness objectives in a safe and progressive manner. Please allow us to encourage your exercise efforts, and to assist you in overcoming strength plateaus. As you become better acquainted with our instructional staff, you should find that they are capable and caring individuals who can make your personal training program a more positive and reinforcing experience.

Whenever you need more motivation, you may schedule an exercise redesign meeting with an instructor, join a high-intensity training session, or participate in our personal training program. You are also welcome to take advantage of our 10-week strength training classes held in our research center with two instructors and six participants per class.

Just let us know how we can better serve you, and we will certainly do our best to make each exercise session the best part of your day.

In addition to the brochure on our management philosophy, we provide a new member training booklet that reinforces the exercise principles and training procedures presented in our orientation slide show. In case you would like to incorporate this information, the strength-related sections of our *All About Exercise* booklet are as follows:

Dear New YMCA Member:

Thank you for attending the South Shore YMCA New Member Orientation Slide Show Presentation and participating in our New Member Training Program.

Enclosed is your training information packet for starting a safe, sensible, and successful exercise program. After reading this material, you will train with an experienced Nautilus instructor who will teach you step-by-step how to best improve your physical fitness.

We wish you much success in achieving your health and fitness goals through planned, progressive, and personally satisfying exercise experiences.

Wayne L. Westcott, Ph.D.　　Claudia Westcott　　Rita La Rosa Loud
Fitness Research Director　　Nautilus Director　　Associate Fitness Director

New Member Training

Program Requirements

1. Attend slide show presentation.
2. Complete medical history questionnaire, and, if necessary, provide medical clearance.
3. Read educational material.
   - How We Manage Our Nautilus Facility
   - All About Exercise

4. Participate in one-on-one training sessions with Nautilus instructor.

Program Recommendations

1. Schedule body composition analysis or full fitness evaluation.
2. Complete evaluation of New Member Training Procedures.

Strength Training

Research during the last several years has clearly demonstrated that regular physical exercise of sufficient intensity and duration can produce remarkable adaptations in the musculoskeletal system. Beneficial physiological changes take place in the muscles, tendons, bones, and even the heart. There appears to be an all-or-none law that triggers these physiological developments.

The three components necessary for musculoskeletal development are:

1. An exercise intensity sufficient to produce approximately 70-80 percent of maximum muscle effort.
2. An exercise duration of about 50-70 seconds per muscle group.
3. An exercise frequency of two to three nonconsecutive days per week.

Although any physical activity that meets these criteria is acceptable, those that isolate individual muscle groups and permit slow, full-range movements, such as Nautilus machines, seem most useful for promoting musculoskeletal fitness.

Sensible strength training for all the major muscle groups results in better body composition, enhanced personal appearance, and the ability to perform essentially all physical activities more easily.

Twelve Reasons to Strength Train

1. Avoid muscle loss.
2. Avoid metabolic rate reduction.
3. Increase muscle mass.
4. Increase metabolic rate.
5. Reduce body fat.
6. Increase bone mineral density.
7. Improve glucose metabolism.
8. Increase gastrointestinal transit speed.
9. Reduce resting blood pressure.
10. Improve blood lipid levels.
11. Reduce low back pain.
12. Reduce arthritic pain.

Strength Training Guidelines

Frequency

Train on an every-other-day schedule. Taking back-to-back strength training workouts is counterproductive because the muscles do not have sufficient recovery or building time. Two training days per week produce about 88% as much strength and muscle gain as three weekly workouts.

Duration

Train with 1 set of 8 to 12 repetitions on each machine. At 6 seconds per repetition a set of strength exercise should take about 50-70 seconds. When the proper weightload is used, this provides excellent stimulus for strength gains.

Intensity

The weightload should be heavy enough to fatigue the target muscle group within 8-12 repetitions.

Speed

Perform all movements slowly, approximately 6 seconds per repetition. Take 2 seconds to lift the weightload, and take four seconds to lower the weightload. Slow training increases the strength building stimulus and reduces the risk of injury.

Range

Perform all exercises through a full range of pain-free joint movement. Full-range training ensures greater muscle effort, joint flexibility, and performance power.

Progression

Gradually increase muscle stress by adding 1 to 3 pounds whenever you complete 12 repetitions in good form. Progressive resistance is the key to continued strength development.

Continuity

Proceed from machine to machine in order and in a timely manner. This works the muscles from larger to smaller groups, and provides better overall training effect.

Recommendations for Safe and Effective Exercise Participation

Consider the following recommendations for maintaining a high level of strength training motivation.

Treat exercise as positive rather than negative.

Most individuals will persist in an exercise program only if it is perceived as a positive experience. This does not necessarily imply that exercise should be easy. What really counts is that exercise effort is something you want to do rather than something you have to do.

Maintain Regular Workouts

Consistency is perhaps the most important variable in developing and maintaining physical fitness. Two or three nonconsecutive workout sessions per week on a regular basis are recommended for maximizing muscular fitness.

Discontinue Your Workout in the Event of Illness or Injury

Be alert to signals that your body is undergoing too much stress, and give yourself time to recover and rebuild. In the unlikely event of the following symptoms *stop exercising and tell an instructor immediately.*

1. Tightness in chest and neck area.
2. Pain or unusual fatigue.
3. Breathing difficulty.

Record important information regarding each training session

Keep a record of each training session on the workout card provided. This serves as a progress chart, a source of motivation and a monitoring system for increasing or decreasing the intensity of your training program.

Wear Specifically-Designed Athletic Shoes and Lightweight Exercise Clothing.

Wearing properly-designed athletic shoes reduces the risk of injury due to slipping or improper transfer of forces. Wearing lightweight exercise clothing reduces the chance of overheating and enhances performance levels.

Drink Plenty of Water Before, During, and After Exercise

Because our muscles are almost 80 percent water, it is essential to be well-hydrated. Try to drink between 8 and 12 glasses of water (or juice) every day for best strength training results.

Wait Two Hours After a Large Meal to Engage in Vigorous Exercise

Waiting two hours after a large meal before engaging in vigorous exercise allows the blood to be channeled to the digestive organs without interference. It also allows food to pass from the stomach, which provides ample room for the diaphragm to move during heavy breathing.

Eat Nutritionally Sound Meals

Proper eating complements the exercise program in terms of lower bodyweight, lower percentage of body fat, lower levels of cholesterol and triglycerides, lower blood pressure, and fewer gastrointestinal problems. It also provides ample energy for your workouts and sufficient nutrients for muscle development.

Implementation Options for the Basic Strength Training Program

Although we sometimes offer the basic strength training program by itself, we generally combine it with aerobic activity, stretching exercise, or both. Our aerobic component is typically treadmill walking or stationary cycling. We begin with an easy effort level and short training duration, then progress gradually to 20 or more minutes of continuous endurance exercise at about 70 percent of maximum heart rate. Our research has shown similar results regardless of whether the endurance exercise precedes or follows the strength exercise (Westcott 1999, Westcott and La Rosa Loud 1999). In other words, aerobic activity performed at a moderate effort level does not seem to interfere with strength development (McCarthy et al 1995). Table 1-4 presents our research results on strength gains attained when endurance exercise is performed before or after strength training. For more information on this research study, please see Chapter 10.

Our flexibility component generally consists of interspersing stretching exercises with the Nautilus machines. We have experienced excellent results by performing a 20-second stretch for the muscle group just worked. For example, the leg extension exercise is followed by a 20-second static stretch for the quadriceps muscles and the leg curl exercise is followed by a 20-second static stretch for the hamstrings muscles. Chapter 2 presents the muscle specific stretches used in our recommended training program, and Chapter 10 provides the results of our studies on combined strength and stretching exercise.

In brief, our recent research has shown that adding stretching exercises to the Nautilus workout may have dual benefits, enhancing both joint flexibility and strength development. As you will note in Table 1-5, the participants who did static

Study	1	2	3	4	Total
Subjects	23	43	71	68	**205**
Assessment Exercise	Leg Extension	Chest Press	Super Pullover	Lateral Raise	**All Exercises**
Endurance Exercise First	+20 lbs.	+9 lbs.	+15 lbs.	+18 lbs.	**+15 lbs.**
Strength Exercise First	+ 23 lbs.	+15 lbs.	+14 lbs.	+18 lbs.	**+16 lbs.**

Table 1-4 Strength gains for major muscle groups with endurance exercise performed before or after strength training (205 subjects).

stretches following the Nautilus exercises had greater increases in hamstrings flexibility (2.4 vs. 1.5 inches) and strength (19.6 vs 16.4 lbs.) than the participants who did Nautilus exercises only. Because our participants typically take a 1-minute break between Nautilus machines, the 20-second stretches did not lengthen the overall workout duration.

Parameter	Nautilus Exercise (n = 36)	Nautilus and Stretching Exercise (n = 119)
Sit and Reach Test* of Hamstring Stretch	+1.5 in.	+2.4 in.
10-Repetition Maximum Leg Curl Test of Hamstring Strength	+16.4 lbs.	+19.6 lbs.
*21 subjects in each group assessed for this parameter		

Table 1-5 Changes in hamstrings stretch and strength resulting from 10 weeks of Nautilus exercise or Nautilus and stretching exercise (155 subjects).

Summary

The basic strength training program is a well-researched and time-tested exercise protocol that has proven safe and productive for muscle development. In agreement with the American College of Sports Medicine strength training guidelines (ACSM 1998), it consists of 12 Nautilus exercises, performed for one set of 8 to 12 repetitions at a moderate movement speed and through a full movement range. At about one minute per exercise and one minute between exercises, the basic strength training program requires approximately 24 minutes for completion.

Adding aerobic activity before or after strength training provides a cardiovascular conditioning component. We have had excellent results with 20 minutes of treadmill walking and stationary cycling. Interspersing muscle specific stretching exercises between Nautilus machines appears to enhance both joint flexibility and strength development, without increasing the total workout duration.

We have found similar strength training benefits for participants who perform two or three exercise sessions per week. However, the key to continued improvement is training consistency. By incorporating a basic strength training program that is both effective and efficient, your clients should have little difficulty doing regular strength workouts that reinforce their exercise efforts with progressive muscular development.

Chapter 2

Time-Teasing Alternatives

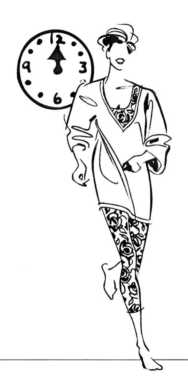

Time-Efficient Strength Program for Time-Pressured People

Endurance exercise, such as jogging, cycling, and stepping, is ideal for improving cardiovascular fitness and for utilizing calories. However, as the name implies, endurance exercise requires relatively long periods of continuous physical activity. The American College of Sports Medicine recommends a minimum duration of 20 minutes for effective endurance exercise (ACSM 1998).

Strength training, on the other hand, can be productively performed in relatively brief time frames. Perhaps the best way to accomplish this is to select a few multi-joint strength exercises that address several major muscle groups simultaneously. For example, the leg press exercise works the quadriceps, hamstrings, and gluteals, the chest press exercise works the pectoralis major, triceps and anterior deltoids, and the compound row exercise works the latissimus dorsi, biceps and posterior deltoids.

Taken together, these three exercises strengthen nine major muscle groups and provide some conditioning benefit to the trunk stabilization muscles (low back and abdominals). Given one minute to perform each exercise and one minute between exercises, the entire strength workout can be completed in about five minutes.

Adult Study With Three Exercises

Can such a short strength training session provide enough muscle building stimulus to produce noticeable results? Based on our research with 59 time-pressured men and women, the answer is yes (Westcott 1992a). This study, known as the *hour per week exercise program*, featured three 20-minute training sessions per week (Monday, Wednesday, Friday) for a period of eight weeks. Of that time, five minutes were used for strength training (3 Nautilus machines) and 15 minutes were used for endurance exercise (stationary cycling or stair climbing). As presented in Table 2-1, the adult program participants made impressive improvements in body composition, lower body strength, upper body strength, and cardiovascular endurance. These included approximately two pounds more muscle, four pounds less fat, 25 percent greater muscle strength, and 12 percent greater cardiovascular endurance. As you might expect, the men and women in the non-training control group experienced essentially no changes (see Table 2-1).

The hour-per-week exercise program took less than half the time of our basic exercise program presented in Chapter One. Nonetheless, the results were pretty impressive, particularly with respect to muscle gain and fat loss. In fact, the abbreviated strength training and endurance exercise protocol proved highly effective in all of the assessment areas.

Brief Exercise Program Protocol

The strength training protocol was identical to the basic exercise program in every respect except for the number of training exercises. The leg press, chest press and compound row were each performed for one set of 8 to 12 strict repetitions. These

Fitness Parameters	Exercise Group (N = 59)				Non-Exercise Group (N = 8)			
	Pre	Post	Change	%	Pre	Post	Change	%
% Fat	25	24	-1	4	23	23	0	0
Fat (lb.)	43	39	-4	10	41	41	0	0
Lean (lb.)	125	127	+2	2	133	133	0	0
CV End (ml)	34	38	+4	12	33	34	+1	3
Leg Strength (lb.)	80	100	+20	25	86	88	+2	3
Arm Strength (lb.)	101	122	+21	21	108	111	+3	3

Table 2-1   Comparison of fitness changes in group that did one hour of exercise per week and group that did not exercise (67 subjects).

exercises were completed with careful attention to technique, emphasizing controlled movement speed (2 seconds lifting and 4 seconds lowering) and full movement range. Whenever 12 repetitions could be completed in good form, the weightload was increased by about five percent (typically 2.5 to 5.0 pounds).

The endurance exercise protocol involved an ascending warm-up period of about three minutes, a steady state training period of about nine minutes at approximately 75 percent of maximum predicted heart rate, and a descending cool-down period of about three minutes. We did not find any response differences due to the exercise order, so we allowed the participants to perform the endurance exercise before or after the strength training according to their personal preference.

It is reasonable to assume that you could substitute related strength exercises without altering the results. For example, the leg press exercise for the quadriceps and hamstrings muscles could be replaced with one set each of leg extensions and leg curls. Likewise, we have experienced similar upper body responses using assisted chin-ups (latissimus dorsi, biceps, posterior deltoids) and assisted bar dips (pectoralis major, triceps, anterior deltoids) in place of chest presses and compound rows. Logically, pulldowns and incline presses should also produce essentially the same upper body training effects.

Of course, other endurance activities such as walking, rowing and elliptical training should result in as much cardiovascular improvement as cycling and stepping. The exercise mode is considerably less important than the training consistency.

Senior Study With Five Exercises

This study was conducted with 19 frail elderly nursing home patients, and will be discussed in detail in Chapter Four on Senior Strength (Westcott et al, 2000). However, these research results are also relevant to this section on time-saving training protocols because the participants did only five Nautilus machines each exercise session. These were the leg press, triceps press, compound row, low back, and four-way neck (which they performed forwards and backwards). The senior men and women (average age 89 years) trained two days a week for a period of 14 weeks. Even though this represented a very low-volume and time-efficient training program, these elderly individuals made significant improvements in muscle strength and body composition. For example, the participants averaged about 80 percent greater leg strength, 40 percent greater upper body strength, four pounds more muscle, three pounds less fat, and 71 percent more mobility distance after the training program.

The senior men and women in this study followed the same training protocol as the basic exercise program, except that they performed fewer exercises. Given their limited physical capacity at the start of the study, the frail subjects found that five Nautilus machines provided a manageable exercise effort and addressed essentially all of their major muscle groups. The leg press strengthened their quadriceps, hamstrings, and gluteals, the triceps press worked their pectoralis major, triceps, and anterior deltoids, the compound row addressed their latissimus dorsi , biceps, and posterior deltoids, the low back targeted their erector spinae, and the four-way neck developed their neck flexor and extensor muscles.

This exercise program helped these debilitated elders hold their heads up, sit without hunching forward, rise from a sitting to a standing position, and walk better. We therefore recommend these five exercises for older or weaker individuals who have problems with posture, standing up, and walking. You will find much more information on senior strength training principles and practices in Chapter Four.

Combined Strength and Stretching Exercises

As you will read in Chapter 10, our recent studies have demonstrated about 20 percent greater strength gains when each Nautilus exercise is followed by a 20 second stretch for the muscles just worked. For this reason, we strongly recommend combining the strength exercises with brief stretches for the target muscles. This procedure produces more muscle strength and joint flexibility, without adding any time to the overall training program. The 20-second stretches fit neatly within the one-minute recovery intervals that most trainees take between successive Nautilus exercises.

Nautilus Expressway Program

The suggested combination of strength, endurance and stretching exercise represents a highly-effective and time-efficient training program for simultaneously improving muscle strength, cardiovascular endurance, joint flexibility, and body composition. For clients who desire a relatively brief but comprehensive exercise experience, we recommend the Nautilus *Expressway* Program that combines 12 standard strength exercises with complementary stretching exercises, along with optional aerobic activity.

The *Nautilus Expressway* strength and stretching exercises are presented in Table 2-2. Given about one minute to perform each Nautilus exercise and about one minute between strength exercises, this part of the training program should be performed within 25 minutes. Adding a 20-minute period of aerobic activity brings the total workout time to approximately 45 minutes. Completing two Expressway workouts a week requires only 90 minutes of total exercise time, yet provides comprehensive conditioning for muscular strength, joint flexibility, and cardio-vascular endurance. Your clients should find the *Nautilus Expressway* to be a safe, effective, and efficient exercise program for improving their overall physical fitness.

Strength Exercises	Stretching Exercises
Leg Extension	Standing Quadriceps Stretch
Seated Leg Curl	Seated Hamstring Stretch
Leg Press	Seated Quad-Ham-Glut Stretch
10° Chest	Seated Chest Stretch
Vertical Chest	Vertical Chest Stretch
Super Pullover	Upper Back Stretch
Compound Row	Row Back Stretch
Lateral Raise	Standing Deltoid Stretch
Preacher Curl	Seated Biceps Stretch
Triceps Press	Seated Triceps Stretch
Lower Back	Seated Erector Spinae Stretch
Abdominal	Seated Abdominal Stretch

Table 2-2   Nautilus Expressway Program*

You will find illustrations and explanations of these strength and stretching exercises in Appendix A.

Brief Strength Training Programs

Based on our studies and experience with time-efficient training, we recommend the following exercise combinations for developing a two-machine, three-machine, four-machine or five-machine strength training program. The strength exercises may be combined with 15 to 20 minutes of aerobic activity for a more complete conditioning session. As previously noted, the endurance exercise may be done before or after the strength training with essentially equal results. We recommend one carefully performed set of each strength exercise, using a weightload that permits 8 to 12 controlled repetitions. One good set of slow-speed and full-range repetitions is a powerful stimulus for strength gain and muscle development.

Two-Exercise Program

In the two-exercise program, the emphasis is upper body strength. This is a brief workout that may be most appropriate for people who already perform aerobic activity such as running, cycling, or stepping.

2 Exercises – 3 Minutes	
Exercises	**Muscle Groups**
Weight Assisted Chin-Up	Latissimus Dorsi, Biceps, Posterior Deltoids
Weight Assisted Bar-Dip	Pectoralis Major, Triceps, Anterior Deltoids

Three-Exercise Program

This program provides strength work for the legs and upper body. It is simple to perform, with three basic exercises for nine major muscle groups.

3 Exercises – 5 Minutes	
Exercises	**Muscle Groups**
Leg Press	Quadriceps, Hamstrings, Gluteals
Bench Press	Pectoralis Major, Triceps, Anterior Deltoids
Compound Row	Latissimus Dorsi, Biceps, Posterior Deltoids

Four-Exercise Program

The additional exercise in the four-machine program places greater emphasis on the shoulder and upper back muscles, thereby providing a more comprehensive upper body workout while still addressing the major muscles of the legs.

4 Exercises – 7 Minutes

Exercises	Muscle Groups
Leg Press	Quadriceps, Hamstrings, Gluteals
Bench Press	Pectoralis Major, Triceps, Anterior Deltoids
Compound Row	Latissimus Dorsi, Biceps, Posterior Deltoids
Overhead Press	Deltoids, Triceps, Upper Trapezius

Five-Exercise Program

Although requiring less than 10 minutes, this five-exercise program gives almost equal emphasis to major muscles of the legs, upper body and spinal column, thereby addressing overall strength and functional posture.

5 Exercises – 9 Minutes

Exercises	Muscle Groups
Leg Press	Quadriceps, Hamstrings, Gluteals
Triceps Press	Pectoralis Major, Triceps, Anterior Deltoids
Compound Row	Latissimus Dorsi, Biceps, Posterior Deltoids
Low Back	Erector Spinae
Four-Way Neck	Neck Flexors, Neck Extensors

Summary

Our research has revealed excellent results from relatively brief exercise sessions. After two months of training just 20 minutes a day, three days a week, 59 adult program participants averaged four pounds less fat, two pounds more muscle, 12 percent greater cardiovascular endurance, and 23 percent more muscular strength. This training protocol involved only five minutes of strength exercise and 15 minutes of aerobic activity. In a study with 19 frail elderly patients, performing five Nautilus machines twice a week for 14 weeks produced four pounds more muscle, three pounds less fat, 80 percent greater leg strength, and 40 percent greater upper body strength, as well as significant improvements in functional ability. The five Nautilus machines (leg press, triceps press, compound row, low back, four-way neck) included most of the major muscle groups, and could be completed in less than 10 minutes. For time-pressured adults, elderly individuals, and people with unusually low fitness levels, brief exercise programs such as these offer productive alternatives to an otherwise sedentary lifestyle. The new *Nautilus Expressway* Program provides an effective and efficient exercise protocol for men and women who prefer brief but comprehensive conditioning sessions that address muscular strength, cardiovascular endurance, and joint flexibility.

Chapter 3

Workout for Weight Loss

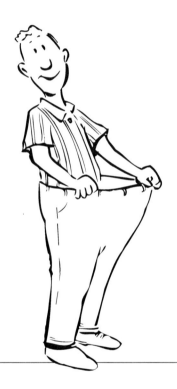

**Strength and Endurance Program
for Winning the Losing Battle**

A 1999 Gallup poll found that 52 percent of all American adults diet in an attempt to reduce their bodyweight (Research Alert 1999). This indicates that one out of two people feel that they weigh too much, and that cutting calories is the preferred means for addressing this problem.

There is no question that most Americans weigh more than they should. In fact, a recent study at Ohio University revealed that nearly 75 percent of the United States population are overweight (Hargrove 1996). However, this finding should be viewed in light of the fact that over 75 percent of Americans are physically inactive (President's Council on Physical Fitness and Sports 1996). It would seem obvious that there is a cause and effect relationship between too little exercise and too much bodyweight.

Unfortunately, the role of muscle in maintaining desirable bodyweight is not understood by most adults. Muscle is very active tissue, and uses a lot of energy all day long for cell maintenance. In fact, at rest a pound of muscle requires over 35 calories a day for ongoing remodeling processes (Campbell et al. 1994). Consequently, adding five pounds of muscle increases our resting metabolic requirements by more than 175 calories per day, and losing five pounds of muscle decreases our resting metabolic requirements by more than 175 calories per day.

Muscle loss is a key component in the weight gain experienced by most men and women during their midlife years. Inactive individuals lose about five pounds of muscle every decade of adult life, resulting in almost a five percent reduction in their resting metabolic rate over the same time period. The lower metabolism means less energy is needed on a daily basis, and the calories that previously fueled our muscles are now stored in our fat cells.

To summarize the basic cause of gradual weight gain in sedentary adults, consider the following sequence of events:

- Lack of strength exercise results in less muscle.
- Less muscle results in reduced metabolic rate.
- Lower metabolism results in reduced energy needs.
- Reduced energy requirement results in more calories stored in fat cells.

Although the typical response to weight gain is dieting, this approach has not proven very successful. Even though Americans spend well over 30 billion dollars annually on diet plans, (New York Times News Service 1991), 95 percent of the dieters regain all of the weight they lost within one year (Brehm and Keller 1990). In addition to being unnatural and unsustainable, low calorie diets actually result in muscle loss (about 25 percent of the total weight loss), which further reduces metabolism, and makes it extremely difficult to maintain the short-term weight loss (Ballor and Poehlman 1994).

In recent years, aerobic exercise has received much attention as a means for burning extra calories and reducing fat stores. Certainly, adding a positive activity such as walking or cycling is more reinforcing than taking away a positive activity such as eating normal and healthful amounts of food. However, as good as aerobic exercise is for using energy and improving cardiovascular fitness, it does not address the underlying issue of fat gain due to muscle loss. Unfortunately, endurance training does not replace muscle tissue that has been lost or prevent further muscle loss.

The key to permanent fat loss is strength training that replaces metabolically active muscle and increases calorie needs 24 hours a day, thereby making it easier to maintain a desirable bodyweight. Dr. Ellington Darden's research has indicated that strength training and dieting may be the best way to simultaneously add muscle and lose fat (Darden 1987). Our studies have shown excellent results from a combination of strength and endurance training, especially in conjunction with a sensible nutrition plan (Westcott 1992b).

Weight Loss Studies

Although personal motivation has a major influence on reducing bodyweight, the following studies may shed some light on the roles of strength training, endurance exercise and diet on the weight loss process.

Study One:
Role of Strength Exercise in Weight Loss Program

The main purpose of our first study was to examine the role of strength exercise in a weight loss program. One group of 22 subjects (Group A) followed the American Heart Association low-fat diet guidelines (20 percent fats, 20 percent proteins, 60 percent carbohydrates), and did 30 minutes of endurance exercise, three days a week for eight weeks. Group A lost four pounds of fat for a four-pound improvement in their body composition.

Another group of 50 subjects (Group B) followed the same American Heart Association low-fat diet guidelines, but performed 15 minutes of endurance exercise and 15 minutes of strength exercise, three days a week for eight weeks. Group B lost 10 pounds of fat and gained two pounds of muscle for a 12-pound improvement in their body composition.

These results, presented graphically in Figure 3-1 on page 26, clearly demonstrate that adding strength training to endurance exercise and diet is advantageous for concurrently increasing muscle mass and decreasing fat weight. While both groups reduced bodyweight, only the subjects who did strength exercise replaced muscle, which may be one reason they experienced greater fat loss. Of course, dietary factors have a major influence on fat loss, and this study did not monitor the subjects' food intake or compliance with the prescribed eating guidelines.

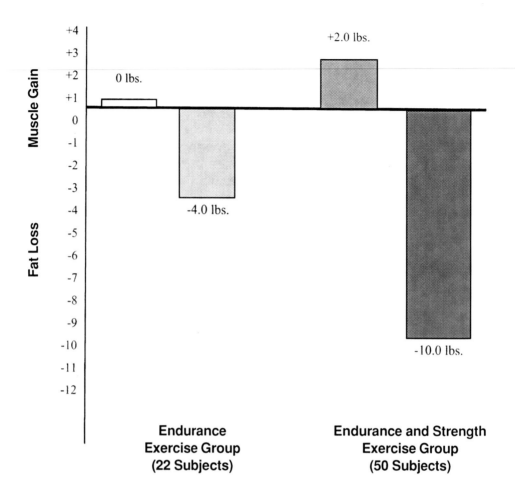

Figure 3-1

Study Two: Role of Diet in Weight Loss Program

The main purpose of our second study was to examine the role of diet in a weight loss program. One group of 61 subjects (Group C) did 25 minutes of endurance exercise and 25 minutes of strength exercise, three days a week for eight weeks. They did not follow a diet plan. Group C lost six pounds of fat and gained three pounds of muscle for a nine-pound improvement in their body composition.

Another group of 90 subjects (Group D) also performed 25 minutes of endurance exercise and 25 minutes of strength exercise, three days a week for eight weeks. However, these subjects followed the Nautilus diet, a low-fat, descending-calorie nutrition plan (Darden 1987). Group D lost 9.5 pounds of fat and gained 3.5 pounds of muscle for a 13-pound improvement in their body composition.

The results of this study (presented graphically in Figure 3-2) suggest that a sensible diet plan may enhance fat loss without diminishing muscle gain. They also

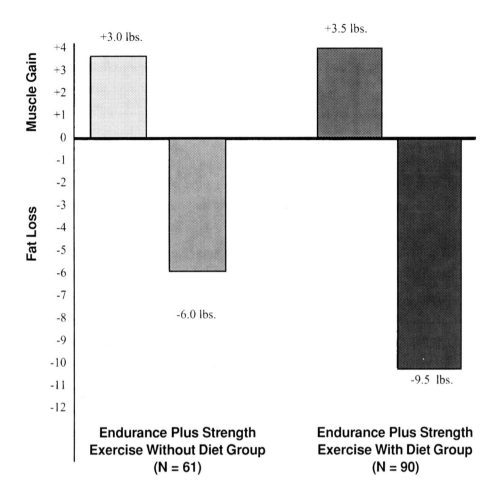

Figure 3-2

support the findings of the first study, that fat loss and muscle gain may occur simultaneously during a sound program of diet, endurance exercise and strength training.

Perhaps the most important outcome of the second study was the participants' response to a written questionnaire administered at the conclusion of the training sessions. All 151 participants reported that they were pleased with the weight loss program, and approximately 90 percent continued to exercise after completing the study.

In summary, these studies indicate that clients attain better weight loss results when strength exercise and dietary guidelines are part of the program. Strength training adds muscle which increases calorie utilization, and a sensible diet decreases calorie consumption. When combined with endurance exercise, this appears to be a productive program for losing weight and improving body composition, as well as for enhancing physical fitness.

Weight Loss Program

Based on these findings, we designed a program that encourages weight loss through a combination of basic strength and endurance exercise. We also provide fairly comprehensive information on healthy nutrition and sensible dieting through weekly in-class presentations.

The strength exercise is our standard Nautilus training protocol, incorporating one set of 12 basic Nautilus exercises. Each set is performed for eight to 12 repetitions at a slow movement speed (six seconds per repetition) and through a full pain-free movement range. The weightload is increased by less than five percent when 12 repetitions can be completed with proper form. The 12 strength exercises and target muscle groups are presented in Table 3-1.

The endurance exercise is a basic program of stationary cycling and treadmill walking, that begins at the participant's present fitness level and progresses gradually to 25 minutes of continuous aerobic activity. We use a warm-up, steady-state and cool-down protocol that does not elicit more than *75 percent of maximum predicted heart rate* or *moderate effort level on the Borg scale of perceived exertion.* Although we attempt to alternate between walking and cycling for cross-training purposes, some participants (such as those with poor balance, orthopedic problems, or excessive bodyweight) are limited to cycling until they are able to safely perform unsupported exercise.

Nautilus Exercise	Major Muscle Groups
Leg Extension	Quadriceps
Leg Curl	Hamstrings
Leg Press	Quadriceps, Hamstrings, Gluteals
Chest Cross	Pectoralis Major
Super Pullover	Latissimus Dorsi
Lateral Raise	Deltoids
Biceps Curl	Biceps
Triceps Extension	Triceps
Low Back	Erector Spinae
Abdominal	Rectus Abdominis
Neck Flexion	Neck Flexors
Neck Extension	Neck Extensors

Table 3-1   Nautilus exercises and muscle groups addressed in the South Shore YMCA weight loss program.

Our research has revealed no response differences whether the strength training is performed before or after the endurance exercise (Westcott and La Rosa Loud 1999). We therefore permit participants to order their strength and endurance activities according to personal preference.

Class Format

To facilitate a high level of instruction, supervision, and motivation, we limit our weight loss classes to six participants with two instructors. Typically, three class members do their endurance exercise while the other three do their strength training, switching activities after about 25 minutes. One day each week, the final 15 minutes of class are devoted to a nutrition lecture with practical props, nutritional charts, and handout materials that provide detailed information on the specific topic being discussed. During the 10-week weight loss program, a variety of nutrition areas are addressed, and class members are provided sample menu plans of 1600, 2200, or 2800 calories per day based on the United States Department of Agriculture Food Guide Pyramid (see Appendix B). Also, each participant prepares a heart-healthy dish that is shared in a culminating pot luck event and included in our members' recipe booklet. Table 3-2 presents our schedule of nutrition lectures and related written materials. Appendix B contains several of our nutrition handouts as samples of written materials that may be helpful to your weight loss program participants.

Week	Nutrition Topic and Handout Materials
1	The Food Guide Pyramid
2	Workout for Weight Loss Menu Plan
3	Carbohydrates – The Base of the Pyramid
4	Protein – How Much Do You Need?
5	Fat – The Good, The Bad, The Deceiving
6	Water – The Most Important Nutrient
7	Facts on Fiber
8	Understanding Food Labels
9	Facts About Fat Substitutes
	Soy Products
10	Healthy Shopping Tips
	Healthy Snacking

Table 3-2   Nutrition topics and related written materials presented weekly in the weight loss program.

Participant Motivation

Most overweight individuals have experimented with different diet programs, but few have had much experience in the area of exercise. This is particularly true for strength exercise, due to the widespread misconception that strength training increases bodyweight. We therefore place a priority on motivating our weight loss program participants through positive and productive exercise sessions. Towards this end, our instructors strive to incorporate the following teaching guidelines during their classes (Westcott 1995a).

1. Clear Training Objectives

The first priority in each class session is to tell the participants exactly what you expect them to accomplish during their workout. For example, "Mary, today I would like you to perform a new exercise, the rotary torso machine."

2. Concise Instruction and Precise Demonstration

Be sure to clearly describe and model the desired exercise technique so there is no confusion on the part of the participant. For example, "Mary, see how my hips stay stationary as I slowly turn my torso about 30 degrees to the left."

3. Attentive Supervision

Even after observing you demonstrate proper technique, many previously sedentary class members lack confidence in their physical ability and prefer not to perform the exercise on their own. Always watch them make their first attempt, as instructor observation is a powerful motivating factor for most new exercisers. For example, "Mary, I will watch you as you try the rotary torso exercise."

4. Appropriate Assistance

To assure proper exercise performance, it is sometimes necessary to provide some form of manual assistance to the participant. For example, "Mary, I will guide you through the first repetition to help you establish the exercise range of movement."

5. One Task At A Time

Discussing more than one performance task may be confusing to new exercisers. Give only one directive at a time to increase the probability of successfully completing each task. For example, "Mary, just concentrate on holding your hips still as you slowly turn your torso."

6. Gradual Progression

It is essential to progress in small steps when instructing people who have little exercise experience. Never introduce a follow-up task until the first task has been mastered. For example, "Mary, your next step is to keep your shoulders square as you slowly turn your torso."

7. Positive Reinforcement

Because new exercisers typically experience some uncertainty about their physical performance, give them positive reinforcement in the form of affirming comments or personal compliments. For example, "Great job, Mary. You did that just right."

8. Specific Feedback

Positive reinforcement is more meaningful when it is combined with specific information feedback. Telling participants precisely what they are doing well increases the likelihood that they will repeat proper technique. For example, "Great job, Mary. You turned your torso without twisting your shoulders."

9. Careful Questioning

Lack of experience may make it difficult for new exercisers to volunteer information that could be useful in designing their training program or refining their exercise technique. Be sure to ask specific questions that elicit informative responses. For example, "Mary, where do you feel the effort as you perform this exercise?"

10. Pre and Post Exercise Dialogue

See if you can sandwich each participant's exercise experience between an arriving and departing dialogue. Taking a minute before and after each workout to engage the member in relevant conversation is time well spent. For example, "Mary, congratulations on learning the rotary torso machine. Please tell me your impressions of this new midsection exercise."

Summary Of Weight Loss Program Specifics

Our Nautilus Weight Loss Program recently received a NOVA 7 Award from *Fitness Management Magazine* for excellence in exercise programming (Martinez 1999). While much credit for the success of this program goes to the inspirational instructional staff and cooperative class participants, specific information about our philosophy, design, and operational procedures may be useful to you.

The primary goal of the Nautilus Weight Loss Program is to provide overweight individuals with practical tools to establish a lifetime commitment to healthy eating and exercise habits. To achieve this, the program includes relevant nutritional information and supervised exercise sessions. The dietary recommendations are made by staff members with four-year college degrees in nutrition and are approved by a nationally-recognized registered dietitian. The educational component consists of 15-minute *Healthy Eating* presentations during the Wednesday classes that address the food guide pyramid, menu planning, food labels, sensible snacking, and a variety of other topics. Each participant also receives weekly menu plans for eating well-balanced meals totaling 1600, 2200, or 2800 calories per day based on the food guide pyramid.

The exercise recommendations are consistent with the American College of Sports Medicine's training guidelines for strength, flexibility and endurance exercise (ACSM 1998). Class members perform one set each of 12 Nautilus machines followed by a 20-second static stretch for the muscle group just worked, which typically takes about 25 minutes for completion. They also progress to about 25 minutes of continuous aerobic activity (treadmill walking or cycling), for a total training time of approximately 50 minutes per session.

Classes are offered on Mondays, Wednesdays and Fridays, at 6 am, 7 am, 8 am, 9 am, 10 am, 11 am, 12 noon, 1 pm, 3 pm, 4 pm, 6 pm, 7 pm, and 8 pm. The program is 10 weeks in length and is available during the fall, winter, spring and summer seasons. Each class is held in a separate, fully-equipped exercise room, and consists of six participants with two instructors for personal instruction and careful supervision. Large attendance sheets are posted to encourage exercise adherence, and members record all of their training information on personal workout cards to facilitate proper exercise progression.

The Nautilus Weight Loss Program averages about 80 members per session, which totals about 320 participants per year. The program fee is $250 per person, which provides about $80,000 in annual income. Also, approximately 70 percent of those who complete the program join the YMCA and continue to train in our large Nautilus Fitness Facility, which adds about 225 full memberships every year.

All Nautilus Weight Loss Program participants must complete a medical history questionnaire (with physician guidelines if necessary), and a fitness assessment including bodyweight, body composition, resting blood pressure, muscle strength, and joint flexibility. After 10 weeks of training, the class members are reassessed in all of the fitness parameters, and consistently show significant improvements in body composition, resting blood pressure, muscle strength, and joint flexibility. Most of the men and women gain two to four pounds of muscle and lose six to 12 pounds of fat, for a major improvement in physical appearance. As a result of their satisfaction with the program, our class evaluations have averaged 4.9 on a 5.0 – point scale. According to the participants, the small class format featuring strength training, flexibility exercise, aerobic activity, nutrition education, and member motivation provides an enjoyable conditioning experience that enables them to look better, feel better, and function better (Westcott 1999).

Cellulite Reduction Program

We have recently introduced a more specialized, supervised and time-efficient training program to address a pervasive problem among women, commonly called cellulite. Cellulite is essentially fat that is no longer evenly distributed under the skin, but is clumped in uneven bundles giving a rippled and dimpled appearance. The most likely cause of cellulite is the combined effects of muscle loss (about five pounds per decade) and fat gain (about 15 pounds per decade). When there is too little muscle to maintain shape, and too much fat for even distribution, the skin takes on the lumpy look of irregular fat deposits.

Cellulite is not a cosmetic problem, so it does not respond to chemical solutions. We believe that cellulite can best be eliminated through a program that replaces muscle and reduces fat. Our approach is a brief program of strength and endurance exercise. Strength exercise builds a firm muscle foundation that facilitates an even fat layer and taught skin, as well as a faster metabolic rate that burns additional calories all day long. Endurance exercise requires high energy expenditure that assists in calorie utilization and fat loss.

Basic Program

The basic strength program consists of five Nautilus exercises, performed for one set of 10 to 15 repetitions at a slow movement speed and through a full movement range. All of the exercises address the hip and thigh muscles, where the cellulite problem is typically most prevalent. The Nautilus machines are the seated leg curl, leg extension, hip adduction, hip abduction, and leg press, and this strength workout require about 10 minutes for completion.

The basic endurance program involves 10 minutes of continuous exercise on a treadmill, cycle, stepper, etc., including about two minutes of warm-up and two minutes of cool-down. We recommend training at approximately 70 percent of maximum heart rate, which corresponds to a moderate effort level.

The combined program takes 20 minutes, and is performed three days per week for a period of eight weeks. Each participant works one-on-one with a personal trainer, who provides high levels of supervision and encouragement throughout the training session.

Extended Program

The extended program adds five more exercises for the upper body and midsection muscles, and requires about 20 minutes for completion of the strength component. The recommended additional Nautilus machines are the bench press, compound row, overhead press, abdominal, and low back.

The extended program also progresses to 20 minutes of continuos endurance exercise, using one or more of the training modalities (treadmill, cycle, stepper, etc.). The total training time for the extended workout is approximately 40 minutes per session.

Program Results

The subjects in our first two cellulite reduction research studies were 23 women between 26 and 66 years of age who wanted to reduce the cellulite on their thighs. They trained at their preferred workout time with a personal trainer on Mondays, Wednesdays and Fridays for a period of eight weeks. Most of the women progressed to the extended exercise program as they experienced positive training outcomes.

On average, the women added 2.0 pounds of muscle and lost 3.3 pounds of fat, for a 5.3-pound improvement in their body composition. They also decreased their hip size by 1.3 inches, and increased their leg strength by more than 60 percent. Thirty percent of the participants reported less cellulite and 70 percent reported a lot less cellulite. This was confirmed by our ultrasound measurements of their thighs, which showed a 1.4 mm reduction in the fat layer and a 1.7 mm increase in the muscle layer. All of the women reported that the exercise program was a positive and productive experience that improved their muscle strength, cardio-vascular endurance, and joint flexibility in a safe, effective and efficient manner.

Although the women would have undoubtedly attained even better results if they followed a reduced calorie diet plan, the brief exercise program produced impressive improvements in their body composition and physical appearance. Perhaps most important, the participants were very pleased with the training outcomes, and indicated that the short sessions and personal supervision were key factors in their decision to join and continue the exercise program.

Summary

By following a program of strength training and cardiovascular exercise, the problem of too little muscle and too much fat can be effectively addressed. Strength training burns calories during and after the exercise session, as well as replaces muscle which uses calories all day long for tissue maintenance. It would also appear that cellulite can be reduced as new muscle helps to restore shape by providing a firm underlying foundation that lessens the lumpy look of irregular fat deposits. Cardiovascular exercise helps to burn calories, which also contrib-utes to a reduced fat layer and a more smooth appearance of the skin.

Chapter 4

Senior Strength

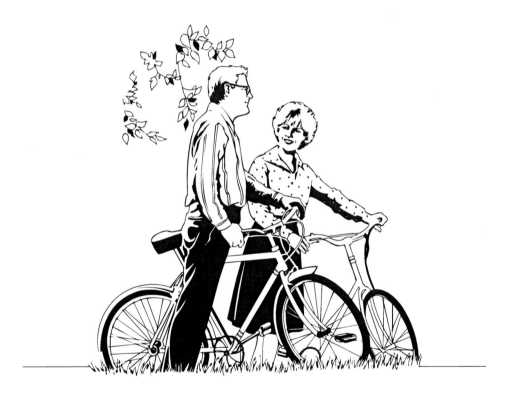

Functional Strength for Older Adults

Perhaps the fastest growing aspect of the fitness field is strength training for seniors, and for very good reason. In fact, in our promotional articles we present over a dozen health-related benefits of sensible strength training. While these reasons may not be motivating for teenagers, they have a profound positive impact on health-conscious older adults. Consider sharing the following research-based reasons for participating in a sensible program of strength exercise with the 50-plus population in your service area.

Reasons for Strength Training

1. Avoid Muscle Loss

Adults who do not strength train lose between 5 and 7 pounds of muscle every decade (Forbes 1976, Evans and Rosenberg 1992). Although endurance exercise improves our cardiovascular fitness, it does not prevent the loss of muscle tissue. Only strength exercise maintains our muscle mass and strength throughout our mid-life and senior years.

2. Avoid Metabolic Rate Reduction

Because muscle is very active tissue, muscle loss is accompanied by a reduction in our resting metabolism. Research information indicates that the average adult experiences a 2 to 5 percent reduction in metabolic rate every decade of life (Evans and Rosenberg 1992, Keyes et al, 1973). Because regular strength exercise prevents muscle loss, it also enables us to avoid the accompanying decrease in resting metabolic rate.

3. Increase Muscle Mass

Because most adults do not perform strength exercise, they need to first replace the muscle tissue that has been lost through inactivity. Although endurance exercise is highly effective for improving cardiovascular fitness, it does not maintain or increase muscle mass. Fortunately, research shows that a standard strength training program can replace about 3 pounds of muscle over an eight-week training period (Westcott 1995b). This is the typical training response for men and women who do 25 minutes of Nautilus strength exercise, just two or three days per week.

4. Increase Metabolic Rate

Research reveals that adding 3 pounds of muscle increases our resting metabolic rate by 7 percent, and our daily calorie requirements by 15 percent (Campbell et al. 1994). At rest, a pound of muscle requires more than 35 calories per day for tissue maintenance, and during exercise muscle energy utilization increases dramatically. Adults who replace muscle through sensible strength exercise have higher energy requirements and use more calories all day long, thereby reducing the likelihood of fat accumulation.

5. Reduce Body Fat

Researchers at Tufts University found that strength exercise led to 4 pounds of fat loss after three months of training, even though the subjects were eating 15 percent more calories per day (Campbell et al. 1994). That is, a basic strength training program resulted in 3 pounds more muscle, 4 pounds less fat, and 370 more calories per day food intake for the senior participants. This represents a triple body composition benefit resulting from strength exercise that is not possible with other types of training

6. Increase Bone Mineral Density

The effects of progressive resistance exercise are similar for muscle tissue and bone tissue. The same training stimulus that increases muscle myoproteins also increases bone collagen proteins and mineral content. Menkes and many other researchers have demonstrated significant increases in the bone mineral density of older adults after just a few months of strength exercise (Menkes et al. 1993).

7. Improve Glucose Metabolism

Researchers at the University of Maryland have reported a 23 percent increase in glucose uptake after just four months of strength training (Hurley 1994). Because poor glucose metabolism is associated with adult onset diabetes, improved glucose metabolism may reduce the risk of this devastating disease. Of course, a better glucose metabolism also results in enhanced energy utilization for improved performance in essentially all physical activities.

8. Increase Gastrointestinal Transit Speed

A study by Koffler showed a 56 percent increase in gastrointestinal transit speed after three months of regular strength training (Koffler et al. 1992). This is significant due to the fact that delayed gastrointestinal transit time is a risk factor for colon cancer. Although more research on this topic should be forthcoming, it would appear that regular strength exercise may reduce the risk of colon cancer.

9. Reduce Resting Blood Pressure

Strength training alone has been shown to significantly reduce resting blood pressure in hypertensive subjects (Harris and Holly 1987). One large-scale study revealed that combining strength and aerobic exercise may be an even more effective means for improving blood pressure readings (Westcott and Guy 1996). After two months of combined strength and endurance training, the 785 program participants dropped their systolic blood pressure by 5 mm Hg and their diastolic blood pressure by 3 mm Hg.

10. Improve Blood Lipid Levels

Although the effects of strength training on blood lipid levels are not fully understood, at least two studies have revealed better blood lipid profiles after several weeks of strength exercise (Stone et al. 1982, Hurley et al. 1988). It is important to note that strength training produces at least as much improvement in blood lipid levels as endurance exercise (Hurley 1994).

11. Reduce Low Back Pain

Years of research on strength training and back pain conducted at the University of Florida Medical School have shown that strong low-back muscles are less likely to be injured than weaker low-back muscles. A recent study by Risch and associates found that low-back patients had significantly less back pain after 10 weeks of specific (full-range) strength exercise for the trunk extensor muscles of the lumbar spine (Risch et al. 1993). Because 80 percent of Americans experience low-back problems, it is advisable for all adults to strengthen their low-back muscles properly. Strong low-back muscles may be the best single measure for preventing low-back pain.

12. Reduce Arthritic Pain

According to a recent edition of the Tufts University Diet and Nutrition Letter, sensible strength training eases the pain of both osteoarthritis and rheumatoid arthritis (Tufts 1994). This is good news, because most men and women who suffer from arthritis pain need strength exercise to develop stronger muscles, bones, and connective tissue. Strength training therefore provides dual benefits, increasing joint function and decreasing arthritic pain in the process.

13. Reduce Depression

A Harvard University study showed that strength exercise is highly effective for reducing depression in senior men and women (Singh 1997). Over 85 percent of the patients who completed a 10-week strength training program no longer met the criteria for clinical depression. This finding indicates that greater muscle strength may be associated with greater self-confidence and a more positive outlook on life.

There are at least 13 physiological reasons to perform regular strength exercise. On a more basic level, it is important to understand that proper strength training may help us to look better, feel better, and function better. Remember that our skeletal muscles serve as the engine, chassis, and shock absorbers of our bodies. Consequently, strength training is an effective means for increasing our physical capacity, improving our athletic performance, reducing our injury risk, and improving our self-confidence.

Small Class Format

Like our strength training program for overweight individuals, we prefer a small class format for our older adult participants. Our 10-week senior exercise program consists of six-person classes with two instructors. Each class involves about 25 to 30 minutes of strength training (12 Nautilus exercises) and 20 to 25 minutes of aerobic activity (treadmill walking and stationary cycling). The trainees perform one set of eight to 12 repetitions in each exercise, and increase the weightload by two to three pounds upon completing 12 good repetitions. They use slow movement speed (six seconds per repetition) and full movement range (without pain). Table 4-1 presents the 12 Nautilus exercises and the muscle groups addressed in our senior strength training program.

How do older adults respond to our standard Nautilus strength training program? Very positively. Almost all report looking better, feeling better and functioning better, and over 90 percent of our senior class members continue strength training after completing the two-month program. In fact, our largest research study found that older men and women respond just as well as younger adults to our basic exercise program (Westcott and Guy 1996).

The 1132 participants in this study included 238 young adults (21 to 40 years), 553 middle-aged adults (41 to 60 years), and 341 older adults (61 to 80 years). As shown in Table 4-2, all three age groups began the program with similar bodyweights (172.7 to 179.9 lbs.) and similar percent fat readings (25.6 to 27.2

Nautilus Exercise	Muscle Groups
Leg Extension	Quadriceps
Leg Curl	Hamstrings
Leg Press	Quadriceps, Hamstrings, Gluteals
Chest Cross	Pectoralis Major
Super Pullover	Latissimus Dorsi
Lateral Raise	Deltoids
Biceps Curl	Biceps
Triceps Extension	Triceps
Low Back	Erector Spinae
Abdominal	Rectus Abdominis
Neck Flexion	Neck Flexors
Neck Extension	Neck Extensors

Table 4-1   Nautilus exercises and muscle groups addressed in the South Shore YMCA senior strength training program.

percent). After eight weeks of exercise, the bodyweight and body composition changes were comparable for the three age groups. The 21 to 40 year-olds lowered their bodyweight by 2.6 pounds and their percent fat by 2.3 percent. The 41 to 60 year-olds decreased their bodyweight by 2.0 pounds and their percent fat by 2.1 percent. The 61 to 80 year-olds reduced their bodyweight by 1.7 pounds and their percent fat by 2.0 percent.

Changes in fat weight and lean (muscle) weight were also similar for the three age groups. The young adults lost 4.9 pounds of fat weight and added 2.3 pounds of lean weight. The middle-aged adults lost 4.4 pounds of fat weight and added 2.3 pounds of lean weight. The older adults lost 4.1 pounds of fat weight and added 2.4 pounds of lean weight.

These findings indicated that senior men and women experience similar body composition improvements as young and middle-aged adults in response to a basic program of strength and endurance exercise. It is interesting to note that the older exercisers replaced muscle at the same rate as the younger program participants.

In addition to body composition assessments, 785 of the study subjects had resting blood pressure readings taken before and after the eight-week exercise

	Age		
	21–40 years (N = 238)	**41–60 years (N = 553)**	**61–80 years (N = 341)**
Body WeightPre (lb.)	176.5	179.9	172.7
Body Weight Post (lb.)	173.9	177.9	171.0
Body Weight Change (lb.)	-2.6*	-2.0*	-1.7*
Body Fat Pre (%)	27.2	27.0	25.6
Body Weight Post (%)	24.9	24.9	23.6
Body Weight Change (%)	-2.3*-	2.1*	-2.0*
Fat Weight Pre (lb.)	49.1	48.9	44.7
Fat Weight Post (lb.)	44.2	44.5	40.6
Fat Weight Change (lb.)	-4.9*	-4.4*	-4.1*
Lean Weight Pre (lb.)	127.4	130.8	128.0
Lean Weight Post (lb.)	129.7	133.1	130.4
Lean Weight Change (lb.)	+2.3*	+2.3*	2.4*

Table 4-2   Changes in body weight and body composition for young, middle-aged and older program participants (1132 subjects).
* Statistically significant change (p<.01).

program. As presented in Table 4-3, all three age groups began with similar diastolic blood pressure readings (76.1 to 80.1 mm Hg). However, the systolic blood pressure readings were considerably higher for the 61 to 80 year olds (143.1 mm Hg) than for the 41 to 60 year olds (127.9 mm Hg) and 21 to 40 year olds (121.2 mm Hg).

Although all three age groups recorded significant reductions in resting blood pressure, the senior participants experienced the greatest improvement. Their diastolic blood pressure decreased 3.7 mm Hg, and their systolic blood pressure decreased 6.2 mm Hg. Perhaps most important, the older adult group began the exercise program with a systolic blood pressure above the hypertensive level (143 mm Hg), but ended within the normal systolic range (137 mm Hg).

The results of this large-scale research study should be encouraging news for senior men and women. Consider the following key findings for the 341 older adults who completed the two-month strength-training program.

1. Seniors can safely participate in well-designed and carefully supervised programs of strength exercise, contingent upon their physician's approval.

2. Seniors can reduce their body weight and improve their body composition. The older adults in this exercise program decreased their bodyweight by 1.7 pounds and improved their body composition by 2.0 percent.

3. Seniors can decrease their fat weight and increase their lean (muscle) weight. The senior subjects in this study lost 4.1 pounds of fat and added 2.4 pounds of muscle after just two months of training.

4. Seniors can reduce their resting blood pressure. The senior participants in this exercise program experienced a 3.7 mm Hg decrease in their diastolic blood pressure and a 6.2 mm Hg decrease in their systolic blood pressure.

Age	Systolic BP Pre (mm Hg)	Systolic BP Post (mm Hg)	Systolic BP Change (mm Hg)	Diastolic BP Pre (mm Hg)	Diastolic BP Post (mm Hg)	Diastolic BP Change (mm Hg)
21-40 years (N = 144)	121.2	116.7	-4.5*	76.1	72.9	-3.2*
41-60 years (N = 375)	127.9	125.4	-2.5*	79.0	76.6	-2.4*
61-80 years (N = 266)	143.1	136.9	-6.2*	80.1	76.4	-3.7*

Statistically significant change ($p<.01$).

Table 4-3   Changes in resting blood pressure for the young, middle-aged and older program participants (785 subjects).

5. Seniors can develop physically active lifestyles, even after decades of sedentary behavior. More than 90 percent of the study subjects continued to strength train after completing the eight-week exercise program.

It would appear that older adults have much to gain from strength exercise, including increased physical capacity, enhanced personal appearance, improved athletic performance, and reduced injury risk. However, many have limited time and energy to participate in a traditional strength-training program. Fortunately, properly performed strength exercise requires a relatively small time commitment. As a case in point, the impressive improvements in body composition and muscle strength experienced by 1132 subjects in the Westcott and Guy study resulted from just two or three brief training sessions per week (Westcott and Guy 1996).

Recommendations For Sensible Senior Strength Training

Several national organizations have developed guidelines for safe and effective strength training, including the YMCA of the USA (Westcott 1987), the American College of Sport Medicine (ACSM 1998), and the American Council On Exercise (Sudy 1991). In general, all of these organizations promote the following program recommendations for sensible strength exercise.

Training Exercises:

The training guidelines call for one exercise for each of the major muscle groups. Table 4-1 presents the standard Nautilus exercises for the major muscles of the body. However, if your clients prefer shorter workouts or a multiple-muscle pushing and pulling exercise protocol, Table 4-4 offers an effective alternative training program.

Nautilus Exercises	Muscle Groups
Leg Press	Quadriceps, Hamstrings, Gluteals
Chest Press	Pectoralis Major, Triceps, Anterior Deltoids
Compound Row	Latissimus Dorsi, Biceps, Posterior Deltoids, Rhomboids
Overhead Press	Deltoids, Triceps, Upper Trapezius
Weight Assisted Chin-Up	Latissimus Dorsi, Biceps, Posterior Deltoids
Weight Assisted Bar Dip	Pectoralis Major, Triceps, Anterior Deltoids
Rotary Torso	Internal Obliques, External Obliques, Rectus Abdominis, Erector Spinae

Table 4-4   Multiple-muscle Nautilus exercises and muscle groups for a shorter senior strength training session.

Training Frequency:

Strength exercise may be productively performed two or three days per week. In terms of strength development, a recent study at the University of Florida found two and three training sessions per week to be equally effective (DeMichele et al. 1997). With respect to body composition changes, subjects in the Westcott and Guy (1996) study who trained twice a week attained almost 90 percent as much improvement as subjects who trained three times a week (see Figure 4-1, below).

Because two and three training sessions per week appear to produce similar muscular benefits, the exercise frequency factor may be a matter of personal preference and scheduling ability.

Training Sets:

Single and multiple-set training protocols have proven effective for increasing muscle strength and mass in senior men and women (Frontera et al. 1988, Fiatarone et al. 1990, Nelson et al. 1994, Westcott and Guy 1996, Westcott et al. 1996). However, studies comparing one and three sets of exercise have found no significant developmental differences during the first few months of training (Starkey et al. 1996, Feigenbaum and Pollock 1999). It is therefore suggested that seniors begin strength training with one properly-performed set of each exercise.

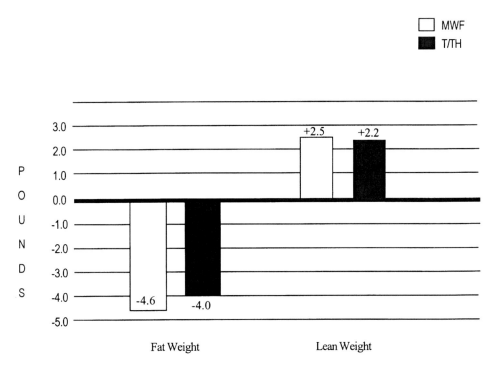

Figure 4-1   Changes in body composition for two and three day per week training groups (1,132 subjects).

This time-efficient approach to strength exercise is safe, effective and well-received by senior men and women. In addition, single-set strength training is very easy for seniors to understand and implement, which appears to be an important factor from a motivational perspective.

Training Resistance

There is a range of training weightloads, generally between 60 to 90 percent of maximum resistance, that is productive for developing muscle size and strength. Weightloads below 60 percent of maximum are relatively light and provide less muscle building stimulus. Conversely, weightloads above 90 percent of maximum are relatively heavy and may present more injury risk.

For most practical purposes, training with 70 to 80 percent of maximum resistance represents a safe and effective weightload range. In fact, many of the studies with senior subjects have successfully used 70 to 80 percent of maximum resistance in their training programs (Frontera et al. 1988, Fiatarone et al. 1990, Nelson et al. 1994, Westcott and Guy 1996, Westcott et al. 1996). As these studies have reported no training-related injuries and have demonstrated high rates of muscle development, exercise weightloads between 70 and 80 percent of maximum resistance are recommended for senior strength training programs.

Training Repetitions

Research indicates that most people can perform about 8 repetitions with 80 percent of their maximum resistance, and about 12 repetitions with 70 percent of their maximum resistance (Westcott 1995b). This represents a moderate number of repetitions per set, and requires about 50 to 70 seconds of continuous training effort when performed at a moderate movement speed (6 seconds per repetition). The recommended number of training repetitions for senior exercisers is therefore between 8 and 12 repetitions per set. However, for frail older adults, it may be advisable to begin training with somewhat lighter weightloads that permit about 15 repetitions per set (Feigenbaum and Pollock 1999). The higher repetition protocol adds a margin of safety for seniors with deconditioned muscles, while providing essentially the same strength building stimulus (Westcott and La Rosa Loud 2000b).

Training Progression

Although it is not problematic to train with more than 12 or 15 repetitions, the key to muscle development is progressive increases in the exercise resistance. Therefore, as training continues, it is advisable to add a little weight whenever 12 or 15 repetitions can be completed in proper form. The recommended training approach is to work with a given resistance until 12 or 15 repetitions are performed, then to raise the weightload by five percent or less. For most senior exercisers, this corresponds to about one to three pounds more weight, which in turn reduces the number of repetitions that can be completed. This double-progressive training system gradually increases the exercise demands and reduces the risk of doing too much, too soon.

Training Speed

There is general consensus that older adults should use controlled movement speeds when performing strength exercise. One study showed excellent and almost equal strength gains for subjects training with four-second, six-second, and eight-second repetitions, indicating that there is a range of effective training speeds (Westcott 1994). Because six-second repetitions have a long and successful history, this repetition speed is recommended for senior exercisers. The preferred cadence is two seconds for the more demanding lifting phase (concentric muscle action), and four seconds for the less demanding lowering phase (eccentric muscle action).

However, two studies have demonstrated significantly greater strength gains from very slow repetitions, requiring 10 seconds for the lifting phase and four seconds for the lowering phase (Westcott 1993, Westcott et al. 1999). Although considerably more challenging, the Super Slow® training protocol may be well-suited for serious senior exercisers who want to maximize their muscle development. This training technique is addressed in detail in Chapter 10.

Training Range

Due to age-related decreases in muscle function and joint flexibility, it is important for seniors to develop strength throughout their full range of joint movement. Research has shown that full-range exercise movements are necessary for building full-range muscle strength (Jones et al. 1988). That is, strength gains appear to be limited to the movement range that is trained. For best results, seniors should perform each strength exercise through the complete range of joint movement, working the muscles from their fully-stretched position to their fully-contracted position. However, if any part of the exercise action causes discomfort, the movement range should be abbreviated accordingly.

Training Technique

In addition to controlled movement speed and full movement range, exercise technique is a critical training factor for older adults. Seniors should always practice proper posture when performing strength exercises, with particular emphasis on body stability and back support. To avoid unnecessary blood pressure elevation older adults should breathe continuously throughout every repetition. The preferred breathing pattern is to exhale during the more demanding lifting movement (concentric muscle action), and to inhale during the less demanding lowering movement (eccentric muscle action). Most important, senior strength trainers should never hold their breath (valsalva effect) or hold the resistance in a static position (isometric effect), as these procedures may raise blood pressure to undesirable levels.

Elderly Strength Training Study

We have found that the same strength training principles and procedures that work so well with senior exercisers can also be successfully applied to frail older adults (Westcott et al. 2000). In a recent study at the John Knox Village (Orange City, Florida), 19 elderly assisted living patients (average age 88.5 years) participated in a 14-week strength training program. Almost all of the subjects were extremely weak and confined to wheelchairs at the beginning of the study. However, by the completion of the program the participants made major improvements in all of their fitness parameters. As presented in Table 4-5, the nearly 90-year-old subjects averaged about four pounds more muscle, three pounds less fat, 80 percent more leg strength, and 40 percent more upper body strength. They also experienced increased functional independence. For example, most of the patients spent less time in wheelchairs, one patient no longer used a wheelchair, and one patient left the assisted living program to join her husband in the independent living apartments. Needless to say, these were very impressive and important improvements, resulting from a brief (six exercise) program of strength training.

Parameter	Pre	Post	Differences	% Change
Bodyweight	130.2 lbs.	131.2 lbs.	+1.0 lbs.	+0.8 %
Percent Fat	22.7%	20.5%	-2.2%*	-9.7%
Fat Weight	29.7 lbs.	26.8 lbs.	-2.9 lbs.*	-9.8%
Lean Weight	100.5 lbs.	104.3 lbs.	+3.8 lbs.*	+3.8%
Leg Press	58.1 lbs.	105.3 lbs.	+47.2 lbs.*	+81.2%
Triceps Press	37.9 lbs.	52.6 lbs.	+14.7 lbs.*	+38.8%
Shoulder Abduction	100.0∞	109.4∞	+9.4∞*	+9.4%
Hip Flexion (Seated)	29.0∞	44.3∞	+15.3∞*	+52.8%
FIM Score	77.5 pts.	88.5 pts.	+11.0 pts.*	+14.2%
Mobility	122.2 ft.	209.4 ft.	+87.2 ft.*	+71.4%
Falls	1.1	0.7	-0.4	-36.4%

* Difference statistically significant ($p < 0.05$).

Table 4-5   Changes in nursing home patients after 14 weeks of strength training (19 subjects).

Based on the findings from this study, the following points may be summarized.

1. Frail elderly can safely participate in well-designed and carefully-supervised programs of strength exercise, contingent upon their physician's approval.

2. Frail elderly can improve their body composition. The participants in this exercise program lost 2.9 pounds of fat and added 3.8 pounds of muscle.

3. Frail elderly can increase their muscular strength. The subjects in this study increased their leg strength by more than 80 percent and their upper body strength by almost 40 percent.

4. Frail elderly can increase their joint flexibility. This strength training program produced about 10 percent improvement in shoulder movement range and over 50 percent improvement in hip movement range.

5. Frail elderly can achieve significant increases in functional capacity. The 14 percent average improvement in *functional independence measurement* experienced by the 19 patients in this program is estimated to reduce their cost of care by about $40,000 per year.

Recommendations for Frail Elderly Strength Training

Our program design and exercise principles for the assisted living patients was identical to that prescribed for our senior strength training participants, with three exceptions. First, due to their initial physical limitations, every strength training session was conducted one-on-one with a physical therapy assistant. Second, the exercise speed was slightly slower, taking about eight seconds for each repetition (four seconds lifting and four seconds lowering). Third, the number of exercises was reduced to six per training session, and specifically selected to improve the patients' functional abilities. As you will see in Table 4-6, these exercises addressed the areas of: (1) overall leg strength (for standing up from a seated position); (2) upper body *pushing* strength (for standing up from a seated position); (3) upper body *pulling* strength (for opening doors and lifting/holding objects); (4) low back strength (for holding the torso erect, allowing better function of internal organs and reducing back stress); and (5) neck strength (for holding the head erect, facilitating breathing, swallowing, speaking, and reducing neck stress).

The length of each exercise session varied between 15 to 30 minutes depending on the level of assistance required by the elderly participants for getting on and off the Nautilus machines. However, their actual activity time was only six to nine minutes per workout as they performed just one set of 8 to 12 repetitions (about 60 to 90 seconds) in the six exercises. They averaged two workouts per week over the 14-week training period. The remarkable improvements in body composition, muscle strength, joint flexibility and functional abilities experienced by these frail elderly men and women clearly indicate that such individuals are extremely responsive to strength training.

Nautilus Exercise	Muscle Groups	Desired Outcomes
Leg Press	Quadriceps Hamstrings Gluteals	Standing up from a seated position, especially getting out of a wheelchair.
Triceps Press	Triceps Pectoralis Major Anterior Deltoids	Getting up from a seated position, especially getting out of a wheelchair.
Compound Row	Latissimus Dorsi Biceps Posterior Deltoids Rhomboids	Opening doors, lifting objects, holding objects, putting on clothes, maintaining proper shoulder posture.
Low Back	Erector Spinae	Holding the torso erect, permitting better function of internal organs, and reducing back stress/discomfort.
4-Way Neck	Neck Extensors Neck Flexors	Holding the head erect, facilitating breathing, swallowing, speaking, and reducing neck stress/discomfort.

Table 4-6   Five essential Nautilus exercises, muscle groups and desired outcomes.

A simple program of six essential exercises, requiring just 12 to 18 minutes of physical effort per week, may be all it takes to make major lifestyle changes in many nursing home patients. Perhaps there is no place where strength training can have a more profound influence on the quality of life.

Summary

There are many reasons that men and women over 50 years of age should perform regular strength training. These include physiological benefits for the muscular system, skeletal system, cardiovascular system, and digestive system.

However, the major advantage of strength exercise is to replace the muscle tissue that is lost at a rate of up to one pound per year in older adults. Regular strength training has been shown to increase muscle mass by more than one pound per month and to increase resting metabolism by over two percent per month, thereby reversing two of the primary degenerative processes associated with aging (Campbell et al. 1994).

Senior exercisers should follow general guidelines for safe, sensible, effective and efficient strength training programs. The basic recommendation for successful strength training experiences are: (1) including exercises for all of the major muscle groups; (2) training two or three non-consecutive days per week; (3) performing one set of each exercise; (4) using between 70 and 80 percent of maximum resistance; (5) performing between 8 and 12 (or 10 and 15) repetitions per set; (6) adding five percent more resistance whenever 12 (or 15) repetitions are completed; (7) using moderate movement speeds, such as six seconds per repetition; (8) exercising through the full range of pain-free joint movement; (9) practicing proper posture; and (10) breathing continuously throughout every exercise repetition.

Research reveals that more than 90 percent of previously sedentary seniors who complete a well-designed, short-term strength training program continue to do strength exercise, indicating that they appreciate the benefits of stronger muscles (Westcott 1999).

Chapter 5

Youth Strength

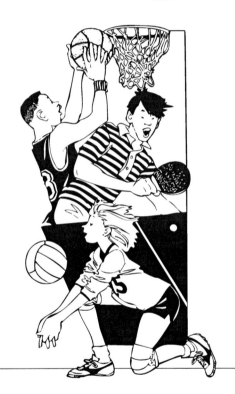

Practical Strength Program for Children

For decades, preadolescents have been prohibited from performing strength exercise because we were led to believe that resistance training would damage their bone growth plates and retard their musculoskeletal development. Fortunately, nothing could be farther from the truth. In fact, there has never been a case of bone growth plate damage due to strength exercise reported in the United States (NSCA 1995). Furthermore, progressive resistance training is the best, and in our increasingly sedentary society perhaps the only way to enhance musculoskeletal development in boys and girls. In fact, a recent study suggested that strength training has its greatest influence on bone formation during the prepubescent years (Morris et al. 1997).

We have also heard that pre-teens cannot benefit from strength training because they do not have enough testosterone (male sex hormone associated with muscularity) to make significant gains in muscle strength. This argument makes no more sense than saying that women or seniors can't increase muscle strength because they have too little testosterone. Obviously, women, seniors, and children can experience major improvements in muscle strength from regular participation in resistance training programs. In a classic study by Faigenbaum and associates (1993), 10 year old boys and girls made overall strength gains of 74 percent after just two months of twice-a-week training (see Table 5-1). Although the non-training control subjects increased strength by 13 percent through normal growth and development, the exercisers made significantly greater improvement (almost six times as much strength gain).

We were then told that training-related strength gains were temporary, and that shortly following the exercise program the children who worked-out would be no

10 RM Strength (in Kilograms)	Exercise Group (n = 14)			Control Group (n = 9)		
	Pre	Post	% Change	Pre	Post	% Change
Leg Extension	12.9	21.2	64.5*	12.1	13.8	14.1
Leg Curl	10.4	18.5	77.6*	12.0	13.6	13.2
Chest Press	15.2	25.0	64.1*	13.4	15.0	12.5
Overhead Press	7.5	14.1	87.0*	7.8	8.8	13.1
Biceps Curl	4.7	8.3	78.1*	4.8	5.3	12.2
Mean % Change			74.3			13.0

* Significant two-way interaction (p<0.01).

Table 5-1   Changes in muscle strength for exercisers and controls after eight week training period (23 subjects, mean age 10 years).

stronger than their untrained peers. A second landmark study by Faigenbaum and associates (1996) proved that this assumption was untrue for the muscles of the upper body. After two months of twice-a-week training, the 10-year-old boys and girls experienced a 41 percent increase in chest press strength. Following two additional months of no strength training the exercise group regressed 19 percent, but was still significantly stronger than the control group in chest press performance (see Figure 5-1). In other words, the strength trained children retained more than half the strength they gained during the two-month exercise period, even after two additional months of no exercise.

Because strength gains have a neuromuscular component, it has been assumed that all strength training improvements in children are due to motor learning rather than muscle development. However, a public school strength training study with 42 preadolescents conducted by Westcott and associates (1995) showed otherwise.

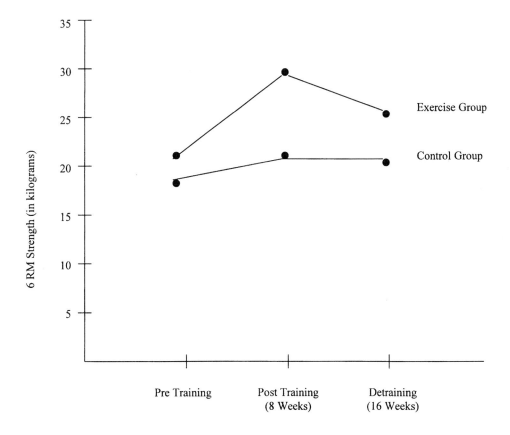

Figure 5-1   Changes in chest press strength for exercise and control subjects over 8-week training and 8-week detraining periods (24 subjects, mean age 10 years).

Group	% Fat Change	Lean Weight Change (lbs)	Fat Weight Change (lbs)
Exercise	-2.7*	+2.5*	-3.0*
Control	-1.9*	+1.5	-1.4*

* Significant change (p<0.01).

Table 5-2 Changes in body composition for exercisers and controls after eight-week training period (42 subjects, mean age 11 years).

As presented in Table 5-2 above, the fifth grade boys and girls who strength trained twice-a-week for eight weeks added significantly more lean (muscle) weight than a matched control group that did not perform resistance exercise. This result indicated that the strength exercise produced muscle development beyond that associated with normal growth in children. The conditioning benefits were so impressive that the children and their parents requested and received a similar strength training program for all of the sixth-grade students the following school year.

Finally, critics have complained that strength training is unnatural and preadolescents don't like doing it. Instead, they argue that young people should exercise with their body weight, doing pull-ups, push-ups and sit-ups.

This has not been our experience at the YMCA or in the school setting. Since Dr. Faigenbaum added classes for repeat participants, we have had many boys and girls sign up for over two years of successive strength training programs. After they outgrow the child-sized equipment, most join a similar program in our YMCA fitness center and continue to strength train on the Nautilus machines.

As noted above, the fifth graders who did strength exercise at school made such impressive physical improvements that they and their classmates participated in an expanded program the following year. Furthermore, 100 percent of the strength program participants reported that it had been a positive experience (Westcott et al. 1995).

So let's summarize what we now know about youth strength training.

1. Strength training does not cause damage to bone growth plates in children.
2. Preadolescent boys and girls can significantly increase muscle strength through progressive resistance exercise.
3. Children who complete an eight-week resistance training program develop and maintain significantly greater upper body strength than their peers, even after an additional eight weeks of no resistance exercise.
4. Preadolescent boys and girls can significantly increase lean (muscle) weight through progressive resistance exercise.

Children typically express satisfaction with both the process and product of supervised strength training.

Bodyweight vs. Progressive Resistance Exercise

Training with bodyweight exercises can be productive if your body is the right weight for your muscular ability. Unfortunately, for most adults and children, our bodyweight is too heavy to permit safe and successful strength development. For example, relatively few adults or youth can perform even one chin-up, making this bodyweight exercise unsuitable for training purposes.

Although not quite as challenging, properly performed pushups present a similar problem for many boys and girls, Let's assume that Johnny can complete 10 good pushups. While this represents an appropriate training load, he is unable to progressively increase the exercise resistance. Yes, he can perform more repetitions with his bodyweight, but adding repetitions is not nearly as effective for building muscle strength as gradually increasing the training resistance.

As for safety, it is far less risky for a child to perform 10 pulldowns on a weightstack machine using half his/her bodyweight (e.g., 40-pound weightstack resistance), than to struggle unsuccessfully with a single pull-up (e.g., 80-pound bodyweight resistance). The major advantage of weight training over bodyweight training is that the resistance can be adjusted to the child's present muscular ability, and progressively increased as strength improves.

With this in mind, let's consider established strength training guidelines for both adults and children.

Strength Training Guidelines

In 1987, the YMCA of the USA became the first national association to publish guidelines for adult strength training (Westcott 1987). A few years later, both the American College of Sports Medicine (ACSM 1990) and the American Council on Exercise (Sudy 1991) issued their recommendations for adult strength training. Fortunately, all three of these fitness organizations presented essentially the same training principles for safe and productive strength exercise. In general, the key training recommendations are as follows:

Exercise Selection: Perform between 8 to 10 basic strength exercises that address the major muscle groups of the body. These include the front thighs, rear thighs, lower back, abdominals, chest, upper back, shoulders, front arms, and rear arms.

Exercise Frequency: Exercise two or three non-consecutive days per week, typically training all of the major muscle groups each workout.

Exercise Sets: Perform one or more sets of each exercise.

Exercise Repetitions: Perform between 8 to 12 repetitions per exercise set.

Exercise Resistance: Use a resistance that fatigues the target muscle group within 8 to 12 repetitions. This generally corresponds to about 75 percent of maximum resistance.

Exercise Progression: Increase the resistance by five percent or less when 12 repetitions can be completed in proper form.

Exercise Speed: Perform each repetition at a controlled movement speed with minimum momentum.

Exercise Range: Perform each repetition through a full-range of pain-free joint movement, from a position of moderate muscle stretch to a position of full muscle contraction.

Exercise Breathing: Breathe continuously throughout every repetition, exhaling during the lifting movements and inhaling during the lowering movements.

These are excellent suggestions for safe, sensible, and successful strength training experiences that can be applied to youth exercisers as well as adults and seniors. However, even before these recommendations were published, the American Orthopedic Society for Sports Medicine, the American Academy of Pediatrics, the American College of Sports Medicine, the Society of Pediatric Orthopedics, the National Athletic Trainers Association, the U.S. Olympic Committee, the National Strength and Conditioning Association, and the President's Council on Physical Fitness and Sports developed a collaborative position paper on strength training for preadolescent boys and girls (Cahill 1988). First presented in 1985 and published in 1988, the updated youth strength training guidelines provide the following directives.

Equipment

1. Strength training equipment should be of appropriate design to accommodate the size and degree of maturity of the prepubescent.
2. It should be cost-effective.
3. It should be safe, free of defects, and inspected frequently.
4. It should be located in an uncrowded area free of obstructions with adequate lighting and ventilation.

Program Considerations

1. A pre-participation physical exam is recommended.
2. The child must have the emotional maturity to accept coaching and instruction.
3. There must be adequate supervision by coaches who are knowledgeable about strength training and the special problems of prepubescents.
4. Strength training should be a part of an overall comprehensive program designed to increase motor skills and level of fitness.

5. Strength training should be preceded by a warm-up period and followed by a cool-down.

6. Emphasis should be on dynamic concentric and eccentric muscle contractions.

7. All exercises should be carried through a full range of motion.

8. Competition is prohibited.

9. No maximum lift should ever be attempted.

Prescribed Program

1. Training is recommended two or three times a week for 20 to 30 minute periods.

2. No resistance should be applied until proper form is demonstrated. Six to 15 repetitions equal one set; one to three sets per exercise should be done.

3. Weight or resistance is increased in one- to three-pound increments after the prepubescent does 15 repetitions in good form.

These recommendations are just as relevant today as they were in 1985, but research studies conducted during the 1990s have enabled us to make a few refinements that enhance both the training efficiency and exercise effectiveness. For example, we recently compared preadolescent strength gains achieved from performing fewer repetitions (6 to 8) with heavier weightloads and those attained from performing more repetitions (13 to 15) with lighter weightloads, over an eight-week training period (Faigenbaum et al. 1999). As presented in Table 5-3, the children who completed 13 to 15 repetitions gained significantly more muscle strength and endurance than those who completed 6 to 8 repetitions. Our findings indicate that preadolescent boys and girls may respond better to training with higher repetitions at lower weightloads than to training with lower repetitions at higher weightloads, at least during the first several weeks of strength exercise.

Variable	Control Group (No Training)	Low Rep Group (6-8 Reps)	High Rep Group (13-15 Reps)
Leg Extension Strength	+13.6 %	+31.0 %	+40.9%
Chest Press Strength	+4.2 %	+5.3 %	+16.3%
Leg Extension Endurance	+3.7 reps	+8.7 reps	+13.1 reps
Chest Press Endurance	+1.7 reps	+3.1 reps	+5.2 reps

Table 5-3   Effects of youth strength training with higher repetitions and lower weightloads vs. lower repetitions and higher weightloads (43 subjects, mean age 8 years).

Our studies also suggest that pre-adolescents who perform one high-effort set of each exercise experience about the same strength gains as those who perform three high-effort sets of each exercise (Westcott and Faigenbaum 1998). In other words, a single set of resistance exercise is an efficient and effective means for increasing muscle strength in young boys and girls. More sets may be performed if desired, but we have not observed much difference in strength development between single and multiple-set training programs in pre-adolescents.

Although young people are prone to doing things quickly, we insist on exercise control achieved through relatively slow lifting and lowering movements. We generally require six seconds for each repetition, with two seconds for lifting actions and four seconds for lowering actions. We believe that controlled movement speeds maximize strength development and minimize injury risk. Because fast movement speeds involve momentum, they may decrease the exercise effect and increase the risk of injury.

Our youth strength training studies have shown similar results from two or three exercise sessions per week (Westcott 1995b). On the one hand, most boys and girls like the strength training program and are willing to exercise three days per week. On the other hand, one or two weekly workouts may make more sense for young people who are involved in additional physical activities such as dance, gymnastics, swimming, tennis, or team sports.

We recently completed a 10-week strength training study with female figure skaters between 8 and 13 years of age (Westcott et al. 1999). Because these athletes skated several days each week, they performed strength exercises just one or two days per week. The younger girls did 10 exercises on child-sized machines, and the older girls completed 10 exercises on standard Nautilus machines. These were, in order, the leg press, incline press, compound row, bench press, shoulder press, triceps press, rotary torso, weight-assisted chin-ups, weight-assisted bar dips, and standing heel raises. All of the participants performed one set of 13 to 15 repetitions, under the supervision of a personal trainer.

Even with the low training frequency, the program participants experienced excellent results. As shown in Table 5-4, the young skaters increased their lower

Parameter	Pre Training	Post Training	Change
Leg Press	47.4 lbs.	94.5 lbs.	+47.1 lbs.*
Bench Press	31.7 lbs.	43.2 lbs.	+11.5 lbs.*
Sit/Reach	19.8 in.	20.9 in.	+1.1 in.*
Vertical Jump	10.2 in.	11.5 in.	+1.3 in.*

*Significant change (p < 0.05)

Table 5-4   Ten-week changes in muscle strength, joint flexibility and performance power for female figure skaters training one or two days per week (16 subjects, mean age 11 years).

Parameter	Pre-Training	Post-Training	Change
Percent Fat	23.3 %	22.3 %	-1.0 %*
Lean Weight	80.2 lbs.	82.7 lbs.	+2.5 lbs.*
Bench Press	34.4 lbs.	49.8 lbs.	+15.4 lbs.*
Sit and Reach	16.9 in.	18.1 in.	+1.2 in.*
Long Jump	54.0 in.	58.8 in.	+4.8 in.*
*Significant change (p < 0.05)			

Table 5-5   Ten-week changes in percent fat, lean weight, muscle strength, joint flexibility and performance power for female figure skaters training one day per week (10 subjects, mean age 11years).

body strength by 99 percent, their upper body strength by 36 percent, their hamstring flexibility by 5 percent, their long jump by 5 percent, and their vertical jump by 13 percent. This latter improvement was most relevant to their skating performance, as the coaches reported much better jumping ability on the ice. Perhaps most important, all of the girls had positive attitudes toward strength training and committed to continue the exercise program.

A 10-week follow-up study was completed using the same exercise guidelines, except that all of the participants trained only one day each week. As presented in Table 5-5, these female figure skaters (8 to 13 years of age) averaged a one-point reduction in percent body fat, a 2.5-pound gain in lean weight, a 45 percent increase in bench press strength, a 7 percent increase in hamstring flexibility, and a 9 percent increase in standing long jump distance, all of which represented statistically significant improvements.

The findings from these studies indicate that a basic strength training program is effective for improving selected fitness parameters and performance factors in female figure skaters. It would also appear that a single weekly session of resistance exercise is sufficient for producing significant strength development in young athletes who are concurrently training and competing in their sport.

Recommended Strength Exercises

The strength workout should ideally address all of the major muscle groups, which may be accomplished by different exercise selections. Table 5-6 presents basic free-weight and machine exercises available on youth-sized equipment that target the major muscle groups. If youth-sized equipment is not available, most children can safely perform strength exercises on standard Nautilus machines that require linear rather than rotary movements. That is, they can do pushing and pulling exercises such as leg presses, bench presses, compound rows, overhead presses, weight-assisted chin-ups, weight-assisted bar dips, pulldowns and

Muscle Groups	Free Weight Exercises	Machine Exercises
Front Thigh (Quadriceps)	Dumbbell Squat Dumbbell Lunge Dumbbell Step-Up	Leg Extension Leg Press
Rear Thigh (Hamstrings)	Dumbbell Squat Dumbbell Lunge Dumbbell Step Up	Leg Curl Leg Press Hip Extension
Inner Thigh (Hip Adductors)	Ankle Weight Adduction	Hip Adduction
Outer Thigh (Hip Abductors)	Ankle Weight Abduction	Hip Abduction
Lower Leg (Gastrocnemius)	Dumbbell Heel Raise	Toe Press
Chest (Pectoralis Major)	Dumbbell Bench Press	Chest Press
Upper Back (Latissimus Dorsi)	Dumbbell Bent-Over Row Dumbbell Pullover	Seated Row Pull-Over Cable Pull-Down
Shoulders (Deltoids)	Dumbbell Lateral Raise Barbell Upright Row	Shoulder Press Cable Upright Row
Front Arms (Biceps)	Seated Dumbbell Curl Standing Barbell Curl Dumbbell Preacher Curl	Preacher Curl Cable Curl
Rear Arms (Triceps)	Standing Dumbbell Triceps Extension	Triceps Extension Cable Press-Down
Lower Back (Erector Spinae)	Bodyweight Trunk Extension	Low Back Extension
Abdominals (Rectus Abdominis)	Bodyweight Trunk Curl	Abdominal Curl
Forearms (Extensors and Flexors)	Bar/Rope Wrist Roll	Cable Wrist Curl Cable Wrist Extension

Table 5-6   Standard free-weight and child-sized machine exercises for the major muscle groups.

triceps presses. However, only those youth who are large enough to align their joints with the machine axes of rotation should perform rotary exercises such as leg extensions, leg curls, chest crosses, pullovers, lateral raises, biceps curls and triceps extensions. Table 5-7 provides our recommended Nautilus machine exercises for boys and girls.

All of our exercisers begin with relatively light weightloads, and progress gradually in small increments (typically one to two pounds). We encourage at least a minute of rest between exercises until the youth increase both their level of fitness and their familiarity with the training program. We also prefer to teach a few basic exercises and systematically add new exercises when the children are ready for more movements.

Before looking at a sample youth strength training class, consider the following summary of our youth strength training guidelines.

1. Select basic strength training exercises that address the major muscle groups of the body. Depending on equipment availability and other factors, this could range from four multiple-muscle exercises to 12 single-muscle exercises, with many variations.

Nautilus Exercise*	Major Muscle Groups
Leg Press	Quadriceps, Hamstrings, Gluteals
Bench Press	Pectoralis Major, Anterior Deltoid, Triceps
Compound Row V (vertical handles)	Latissimus Dorsi, Biceps, Posterior Deltoid, Rhomboids
Incline Press	Pectoralis Major, Anterior Deltoid, Triceps
Compound Row H (horizontal handles)	Posterior Deltoid, Biceps, Latissimus Dorsi, Rhomboids
Overhead Press	Deltoid, Triceps, Upper Trapezius
Weight-Assisted Chin-Up	Latissimus Dorsi, Biceps, Posterior Deltoids
Weight Assisted Bar-Dip	Pectoralis Major, Anterior Deltoid, Triceps

Note: The rotary torso machine is appropriate for most children as the axis of rotation is through the back (spinal column). Including this machine provides resistance exercise for the midsection muscles with emphasis on the internal and external obliques.

Table 5-7   Recommended Nautilus machine linear exercises for boys and girls.

2. Perform 10 to 15 repetitions of each exercise with emphasis on proper technique (slow movement speed, full movement range, continuous breathing).

3. Increase the resistance by a small amount (one to two pounds) when 15 repetitions are completed in good form.

4. Begin with one set of each strength exercise. If 12 exercises are performed use a single-set training protocol. If six exercises are performed, progress to two sets of each with about a minute rest between sets. If four exercises are performed, progress to three sets of each with about a minute rest between sets.

5. Exercise two or three days per week, keeping in mind that both training frequencies appear to produce similar strength gains in youth. Athletes in training may achieve significant strength development with a single weekly workout.

Sample Youth Strength Training Class

Our youth strength training classes are 60 minutes long. We spend about 15 minutes warming up; about 20 minutes performing strength exercises and about 15 minutes cooling down, with about 10 minutes of demonstrations and explanations. Although the warm-up and cool-down segments vary, they always include aerobic activity, stretching exercises and light resistance exercises. The following is a typical class format:

3:15 PM Welcome participants to class. Present class objectives and answer any questions regarding the day's planned activities. Have youth sign in on attendance sheets.

3:20 PM Perform step aerobics with basic movements.

3:25 PM Play the game "Follow the Leader" throughout the exercise area, varying the locomotor patterns.

3:30 PM Perform trunk curls, static and dynamic stretching and three resistance band exercises.

3:35 PM Explain and demonstrate new strength exercises. Distribute workout cards and pencils to record exercise information on class training logs.

3:40 PM Perform strength exercises. (We typically have eight to 12 training stations, with one instructor assigned to every four participants. Participants usually take about 30 seconds to set their seats and weightloads, a minute to complete their exercise repetitions, and 30 seconds to wipe off the machine and record their training information.)

4:00 PM Play a continuous relay game that works different ball-handling skills and locomotor patterns.

4:10 PM Perform static stretching and then wrap up the session by thanking participants by name for their exercise efforts.

Our youth Nautilus strength procedures are similar to our adult exercise protocols with the exception of the repetitions scheme. Because our research indicates that boys and girls make greater strength gains with higher repetitions than lower repetitions, we recommend a two-month introductory training program that begins with 13 to 15 repetitions and progresses to 10 to 12 repetitions. As shown in Table 5-8, we suggest presenting three Nautilus machines during the first two weeks, introducing three more Nautilus machines over the next two weeks, and teaching three additional Nautilus machines over the following two weeks. This

Weeks	Exercises	Sets	Repetitions
1&2	Leg Press	1	13-15
	Bench Press	1	13-15
	Compound Row (vertical)	1	13-15
3&4	Leg Press	1	13-15
	Bench Press	1	13-15
	Compound Row (vertical)	1	13-15
	Incline Press	1	13-15
	Compound Row (horizontal)	1	13-15
	Rotary Torso	1	13-15
5&6	Leg Press	1	13-15
	Bench Press	1	13-15
	Compound Row (vertical)	1	13-15
	Incline Press	1	13-15
	Compound Row (horizontal)	1	13-15
	Overhead Press	1	13-15
	Weight-Assist Chin-Up	1	13-15
	Weight-Assist Bar-Dip	1	13-15
	Rotary Torso	1	13-15
7&8	Leg Press	1	10-12
	Bench Press	1	10-12
	Compound Row (vertical)	1	10-12
	Incline Press	1	10-12
	Compound Row (horizontal)	1	10-12
	Overhead Press	1	10-12
	Weight-Assist Chin-Up	1	10-12
	Weight-Assist Bar-Dip	1	10-12
	Rotary Torso	1	10-12

Table 5-8   Recommended two-month Nautilus strength training program for preadolescent boys and girls.

progressive program of strength exercise instruction encourages good training technique and enhances machine mastery with minimum confusion on the part of the children.

Educational and Motivational Techniques

Although the recommended strength training procedures are relatively simple and straightforward, successful implementation typically requires some instructional and motivational skills. Our youth strength training staff attempt to incorporate the following teaching techniques to encourage purposeful participation and to enhance the exercise experience (Westcott 1995b).

1. Offer a clear training objective for each exercise session.
2. Give concise exercise instructions and precise exercise demonstrations.
3. Provide attentive supervision for all program participants.
4. Give appropriate assistance whenever necessary, and especially with exercise execution.
5. Teach one task at a time.
6. Progress safely and systematically in all aspects of the strength training program.
7. Give plenty of positive reinforcement for good efforts.
8. Provide specific information feedback on exercise performance and training progress.
9. Ask relevant questions to facilitate critical thinking and two-way communications.
10. Welcome each child to class and commend each child for participating in the exercise program during every training session.

Summary

There are few areas in the field of fitness more important than youth strength training. By taking a sensible and serious approach to resistance exercise for children, we can help boys and girls develop both strong musculoskeletal systems and physically active lifestyles that should have lifetime benefits. In fact, recent research indicates that strength training has its greatest influence on bone formation during the prepubescent years. It is good to know that supervised strength training programs for boys and girls have an excellent record with respect to safety and productivity. Our recommended protocol for effective and efficient youth strength training is 8 to 12 basic exercises for the major muscle groups, initially performed for one set of 13 to 15 repetitions, at a slow movement speed and through a full movement range. We also advise that each exercise session include aerobic, flexibility and game activities, as well as relevant fitness information for best overall response and results.

Chapter 6

Strength on the Links

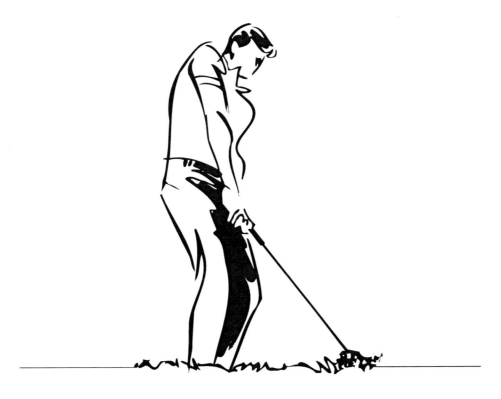

Strength and Flexibility Program for Great Golf

Generally speaking, people of all ages enjoy competitive sports. Unfortunately, as we age, we tend to replace high-energy participation sports (basketball, soccer, tennis, etc.) with low-energy spectator sports (televised football, basketball, baseball, etc.). One exception to the rule is golf, a popular sport played by 25 million Americans, many of whom are middle-aged and older.

Golf is a challenging game requiring much physical skill and often offering hours of time in a beautiful outdoor environment. However, those golfers who do not walk the course experience relatively little physical activity and essentially no cardiovascular or musculoskeletal benefits. Even more problematic, the explosive action of the golf swing places high stress on vulnerable joint structures, including the low back, hip and shoulder areas. In other words, golf is an activity that offers little fitness benefit but carries considerable injury risk.

Due to the length of a typical golf game, many golfers make this their primary physical activity. Others find time to practice on their own or take golf lessons, but the emphasis is skill refinement rather than fitness development. Some golfers are willing to perform a few stretching exercises, as they believe that increased flexibility may enhance their swinging ability. However, few believe that endurance exercise has any relevance to better golf, and most seem to think that strength training will make them tight and less coordinated. In fact, many are fearful that strength training will increase both their body weight and blood pressure, so they deliberately avoid this type of exercise.

Actually, strength training can significantly increase golf driving power, improve body composition and reduce resting blood pressure (Westcott et al. 1996). In fact, strength training can also alleviate low back problems (Risch et al. 1993), and ease arthritic discomfort (Tufts 1994). Clearly, golfers should embrace rather than eschew strength exercise.

Unfortunately, most golfers are unaware of these strength training benefits. Even if they read about a professional golfer who does strength exercise, they typically lack the competence and confidence to start a strength training program on their own.

So what can we do as fitness professionals to change this situation? How can we encourage golfers to participate in a strength exercise program? Our approach focuses on education and motivation.

Educating Golfers

This first step in changing established behavior patterns is education. Golfers are more likely to do strength exercise when they realize that it can improve their playing ability and their physical fitness. Fortunately, there is research data to support these aspects of the educational process.

Consider the results of four separate studies that examined the effects of strength training and stretching on golf driving performance (Draovitch and Westcott 1999). In all studies, the participants were assessed for driving power (club head speed), blood pressure, and body composition parameters before and after the 8-week training period. All of the participants followed a standard program of Nautilus strength training (12 to 16 exercises). Each exercise was performed for one set of 8 to 12 repetitions, using slow movement speed (2 seconds lifting, 4 seconds lowering), and full movement range. When 12 repetitions were completed in proper form, the weightload was increased by one to three pounds.

As you can see in Table 6-1, participants in all four training programs experienced improved body composition and reduced resting blood pressure. On average, the golfers lost 4.1 pounds of fat, added 3.9 pounds of muscle, and lowered their mean resting blood pressure by 4.5 mm Hg. These statistically significant changes were most impressive and highly motivational to the participants.

Although all 77 participants increased their driving power, those who did both strength training and stretching exercises made greater improvements than those who did strength training alone. As you will note in Table 6-2 on the following page, the 25 golfers who performed six stretching exercises on a StretchMate apparatus increased their club head speed twice as much as the 52 golfers who did not stretch (5.2 vs. 2.6 mph).

These findings make sense with respect to the power formula, namely:

$$\text{Performance Power} = \frac{\text{Muscle Force} \times \text{Movement Distance}}{\text{Time}}$$

Variable	1995 (N = 17)	1996 (N = 31)	1997 (N = 21)	1998 (N = 8)	All (N = 77) Age = 57; M = 63, F = 14
Club Head Speed (MPH)	+5.0	+3.0	+1.9	+5.5	**+3.4**
Body Weight (Lbs.)	+1.1	-0.5	-1.1	+0.8	**-0.2**
Percent Fat (%)	-1.6	-2.4	-2.2	-1.8	**-2.0**
Fat Weight (Lbs.)	-3.0	-4.8	-4.4	-3.0	**-4.1**
Lean Weight (Lbs.)	+4.1	+4.3	+3.3	+3.8	**+3.9**
Mean Blood Pressure (mm Hg)	-5.0	-6.4	-1.4	-4.5	**-4.5**

Table 6-1   Results of South Shore YMCA golf conditioning studies (77 subjects).

Strength & Stretch (N = 25)		Strength Only (N = 52)
+5.2 MPH	Club Head Speed	+2.6 MPH
+1.0 Lbs.	Bodyweight	-0.7 Lbs.
-1.7%	Percent Fat	-2.3 %
-3.0 Lbs.	Fat Weight	-4.6 Lbs.
+4.0 Lbs.	Lean Weight	+3.9 Lbs.

Table 6-2   Performance and Body Composition Changes Resulting From Strength and Stretch Training or Strength Only Training (77 subjects).

As applied to golf, driving power may be enhanced by increasing the muscle force, increasing the swing distance, or decreasing the swing time. Strength training is the best means for increasing muscle force, and stretching exercise is the best means for increasing swing distance. That is, muscle strength is the key to producing greater movement force, and joint flexibility is the key to producing greater movement range, both of which have a positive impact on driving power.

Compare changes in club head speed and joint flexibility for two of the golf research groups. Group 1 (1995) did strength training and stretching exercise. On average, these participants experienced a 24-percent improvement in hip and shoulder flexibility, and a 5.0 mph increase in club head speed.

Group 2 (1996) did only strength training. On average, these subjects experienced a 6-percent improvement in hip and shoulder flexibility, and a 3.0 mph increase in club head speed.

Both groups added approximately four pounds of muscle, and increased their leg strength by about 60 percent. Therefore, the greater increase in driving power attained by Group 1 was most likely due to the greater increase in joint flexibility that resulted from the complementary stretching exercises.

Based on these findings we recommend a golf conditioning program that includes both strength training and stretching exercise. Please note, however, that all of the research subjects (strength training only and strength training plus stretching) reported an improved feeling of well-being and better physical function both on and off the golf course. More specifically, the golfers claimed to have longer drives, lower scores and less fatigue during games. Although many of the participants began the program with shoulder, hip or low back pain, none of the golfers reported an injury during the subsequent playing season. This information has proven most helpful in motivating men and women to join our golf conditioning program.

Motivating Participants

We typically provide educational information through various presentations and publications. Presentations to service groups, such as Rotary, Kiwanis and Lions Clubs, are good opportunities to interact with local golfers and answer their questions about strength training, physical fitness and performance enhancement.

In our experience, the best publication for providing exercise information to the golfing community is the local newspaper. We supply a weekly fitness column to the daily newspaper, but articles in weekly newspapers should be just as effective. After periodically reading about the benefits of strength training and the positive results of our golf exercise studies, many golfers are ready for the next step in our educational process.

About two weeks before we begin a new golf conditioning program, the newspaper column summarizes information on strength training for golfers and invites all interested readers to attend an orientation session at our facility. Although this is primarily an educational event featuring a slide presentation and question-answer period, the overall intent of the orientation session is to motivate the attendees into action.

Different things motivate different people. However, we have found that the four most motivational aspects of the orientation session are (1) seeing other interested golfers, (2) seeing the exercise facility and (3) meeting the instructional staff, (4) learning firsthand about the golf conditioning benefits from the program director.

There seems to be security in numbers, and seeing a room full of golfers who are interested in strength training makes people more confident about joining the program. It is even more motivating to have one or two golfers who have completed a previous golf conditioning program present the benefits they experienced in their own words. For example, one of our first golf conditioning participants reduced his body fat from 21 percent to 14 percent, and increased his club head speed from 85 mph to 100 mph after 18 months of consistent training. As a 63-year-old six handicap golfer, he is a superb spokesperson for the positive effects of strength training on personal fitness and golf perfomance.

A tour of the exercise facility can be highly reassuring to the golfers who have never done strength training. Concise explanations and precise demonstrations on a couple of Nautilus machines can reduce intimidation and increase the confidence of potential program participants.

Having the program instructors walk small groups through the facility gives individuals the opportunity to interact informally with their future mentors. This provides a personal touch with name-face association, and assures the new class members that they are joining a high-quality program with competent and caring leadership.

The tours end at the registration desk where extra staff members are on hand to enroll those golfers who want to join the program. Upon registering, the new members receive a welcome sheet with important details about their class dates, times and operational procedures, as well as a medical history form, a personal fitness packet, and a fitness/performance assessment schedule. They leave feeling that they learned relevant information, received personal attention and made a good decision in joining the program.

But motivation doesn't end at the orientation meeting. Each class must be a safe, satisfying and successful experience for the participants to continue strength training, especially during the early conditioning phase. We address this objective with (1) small classes, (2) close supervision, (3) a separate training facility and (4) brief exercise sessions.

We prefer six-person classes with two instructors, as this provides an interactive training community with ample personal attention. We hold our classes in a separate exercise facility to reduce distraction and enhance training focus. If this is not possible for you, consider conducting the conditioning classes during lower-use times in the general fitness center, perhaps on a separate line of machines. Because most golfers tend to have time constraints, we offer brief activity sessions with about 25 minutes of strength training and five minutes of stretching exercise.

Because self-recording is a reinforcing behavior, every participant keeps a detailed workout card, and checks off each training session on posted attendance placards. On average, the golfers make over 85 percent of their scheduled exercise sessions.

Reinforcement also comes from the instructors, who provide positive feedback on those things the exercisers are doing well and encouragement in those areas that are yet to be mastered.

At the conclusion of the program, each golfer is reassessed, and praised for any fitness and performance improvements he or she has achieved. Those who attended more than 90 percent of their scheduled classes receive a t-shirt, and all are given two additional weeks of facility use for completing the program. During this period, many of the class participants choose to continue training on their own and take out a yearly membership.

And this is when all of the work becomes worth the effort. Each golfer who becomes a regular exerciser not only benefits personally, but serves as a model for other golfers to join the next program and attain similar results. The word soon gets around that a basic program of strength and stretching exercise is good for golfers and for their game.

A key motivational component of the golf conditioning classes is the pre- and post-training assessments of club head speed. We use a relatively inexpensive radar monitoring device (Swingmate by Beltronics) available at many golf equipment stores. We also have a small golf net, driving mat and standard golf clubs that we use for the swing-speed assessments. For comparison purposes, we allow each participant to take several practice swings and then average five consecutive best effort drives. This provides an objective measurement of the golfers' improvement in driving power over the course of the training program.

Recommended Golf Conditioning Program

We have had excellent results with a standard program of 12 Nautilus exercises and 6 StretchMate stretches. Our basic golf conditioning program is presented in Table 6-3. All of the strength exercises are performed for one set of 8 to 12 repetitions using slow movement speed (2 seconds lifting, 4 seconds lowering), full movement range, and gradual progression (1 to 3 pound weightload increase upon completing 12 repetitions). All of the stretches are held for approximately 20 seconds in a position of muscle taughtness without discomfort.

Nautilus Machine	Target Muscles	Relevance to Driving Action
Leg Extension	Quadriceps	Power Production
Leg Curl	Hamstrings	Power Production
Leg Press	Quadriceps, Hamstrings, Gluteals	Power Production
Chest Cross	Pectoralis Major	Swing Action
Super Pullover	Latissimus Dorsi	Swing Action
Lateral Raise	Deltoids	Swing Action
Biceps Curl	Biceps	Club Control
Triceps Extension	Triceps	Club Control
Low Back	Erector Spinae	Force Transfer
Abdominal	Rectus Abdominis	Force Transfer
Neck Flexion	Sternocleidomastoids	Head Stability
Neck Extension	Upper Trapezius	Head Stability
StretchMate Exercise	**Target Muscles**	**Relevance to Driving Action**
Front Leg Stretch	Quadriceps	Power Production
Rear Leg Stretch	Hamstrings	Power Production
Hip Stretch	Gluteals	Power Production
Shoulder Stretch	Deltoids, Latissimus Dorsi	Swing Action Swing Action
Back Stretch	Erector Spinae Latissimus Dorsi	Force Transfer Swing Action
Midsection Stretch	Rectus Abdominis Pectoralis Major	Force Transfer Swing Action

Table 6-3 Basic golf conditioning program exercises, muscles, and relevance to driving action.

If more muscle strengthening exercises are desired, we recommend five additional Nautilus machines that have a somewhat sport specific application. These exercises, presented in Table 6-4, have been especially well-received by our golf program participants. We suggest staying with the basic Nautilus exercises for at least four weeks, then adding one or two new exercises per week in the order desired. Just make sure to add or delete exercises in an appropriate manner, so that all of the major muscle groups are addressed each workout, using 12 to 17 Nautilus machines.

Nautilus Machine	Target Muscles	Relevance to Driving Action
Rotary Torso	Internal Obliques,	Force Transfer
	External Obliques	Force Transfer
Hip Adduction	Hip Adductor Group	Power Production
Hip Abduction	Hip Abductor Group	Power Production
Super Forearm	Wrist Flexors	Club Control
	Wrist Extensors	Club Control
	Wrist Pronators	Club Control
	Wrist Supinators	Club Control
Rotary Shoulder	External Rotators	Swing Action
	Internal Rotators	Swing Action

Table 6-4   Additional Nautilus exercises with more golf specific applications.

Summary

Golfers have traditionally avoided strength training for fear of adding bodyweight, developing large muscles, feeling tight, losing speed, compromising coordination, experiencing errant drives and posting higher scores. Fortunately, recent research has proven these perceptions to be false. In fact, just two months of basic strength training combined with six stretching exercises has been shown to improve body composition (4 pounds more muscle and 4 pounds less fat), increase muscle strength (almost 60 percent), enhance joint flexibility (24 percent), and increase club head speed (6 percent). In addition, the strength-trained golfers reported longer drives, lower scores and no injuries during the subsequent golf season. We strongly recommend the 30-minute program of strength and stretching exercise to golfers who want to feel better, function better and play better on the links.

Advanced Strength Training

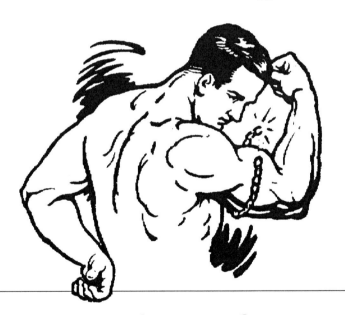

High Intensity Strength Program for Greater Gains

Beginning strength trainers eventually become advanced exercisers, a transition typically signified by attaining strength plateaus in their Nautilus workouts. That is, the standard training procedures fail to elicit further strength gains or muscle development. Generally speaking, strength plateaus indicate a need to redesign the exercise program. Although there are many ways to change the training variables (exercises, sets, repetitions, etc.), we suggest that switching to a high-intensity program may be the most productive approach (Westcott 1996a).

Research and Design for High-Intensity Strength Training

It is well understood that single-set training is highly effective for strength development in beginning exercisers (Feigenbaum and Pollock 1999). However, there is a common misconception that multiple-set training is more productive for advanced exercisers. With respect to training effectiveness, we have no quarrel with multiple-set advocates. However, with respect to training efficiency, we favor a less time-consuming approach known as high-intensity strength training.

Although there are several high-intensity training procedures, they can basically be placed in two general categories. Category one is characterized by techniques that extend the length of the exercise repetition, such as *Super Slow®* training. Category two is characterized by techniques that extend the length of the exercise set, such as breakdown and assisted training. All of these training procedures have proven highly productive in research studies with both beginning and advanced exercisers. In fact, in 1999, 10 of the 30 teams in the National Football League used high-intensity training for their strength workouts. Rather than spend two or three hours a day in the weightroom, professional football players on these teams typically performed two 45-minute total-body strength workouts per week.

Extending the Exercise Repetition

Perhaps the simplest way to increase muscle force output and time of muscle tension is to slow down the repetition speed. As illustrated in Figure 7-1, maximum effort knee extensions and knee flexions produce more muscle force (height of the assessment curves) and more muscle tension (area under the assessment curves) at slower speeds than at faster speeds. It therefore follows that slower exercise movements should provide a better strength-building stimulus. To test this theory we conducted two strength training studies with closely matched beginning exercisers.

Study One: Slow Training

In this study, 74 previously untrained men and women performed one set of 13 Nautilus exercises, three days a week, for eight weeks (Westcott et al. 1999). Half

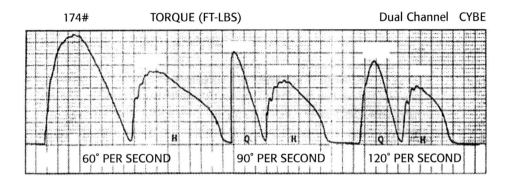

Figure 7-1   Isokinetic assessment of muscle force production at various movement speeds. Muscle force and muscle tension decrease as exercise speed increases.

of the subjects did eight to 12 repetitions per set at the standard speed of seven seconds each (2 seconds lifting, 1 second hold, 4 seconds lowering). The other half did four to six repetitions per set at the slow speed of 14 seconds each (10 seconds lifting, 4 seconds lowering). This protocol, developed by Ken Hutchins, is trademarked as *Super Slow®* training.

At the completion of the study, the standard speed trainees increased their exercise weightloads by 17.5 pounds, and the slow speed trainees increased their exercise weightloads by 26.5 pounds (see Table 7-1). In other words, the slow speed exercisers attained 50 percent greater strength gains than the regular speed exercisers.

Study Two: Slow Training

In this study, 73 previously untrained men and women performed one set of 13 Nautilus exercises, two or three days a week, for 10 weeks (Westcott et al. 1999). Forty-three subjects completed eight to 12 repetitions per set at the standard speed of seven seconds each (2 seconds lifting, 1 second hold, 4 seconds lowering), and 30 subjects completed four to six repetitions per set at the slow speed of 14 seconds each (10 seconds lifting, 4 seconds lowering).

At the end of the training period, the standard speed exercisers increased their chest press strength by 16.3 pounds, and the slow speed exercisers increased their chest press strength by 24.0 pounds (see Table 7-1). As in the first study, the slow speed trainees achieved 50 percent greater strength gains than the regular speed trainees. In both studies, the slow training group developed significantly greater strength than the standard training group ($p < .05$).

	Beginning Weightload	Ending Weightload	Weightload Change
Study 1 Standard Speed	45.2 lbs.	62.7 lbs.	+17.5 lbs.
Study 2 Slow Speed	44.7 lbs.	71.2 lbs.	+26.5 lbs.*
Study 2 Standard Speed	57.7 lbs.	74.0 lbs.	+16.3 lbs.
Study 2 Slow Speed	54.9 lbs.	78.9 lbs.	+24.0 lbs.*

* In both studies the slow speed training produced 50% greater strength gains.

Table 7-1 Changes in muscle strength for standard speed and slow speed exercise groups (147 subjects).

Based on these findings, it would appear that *Super Slow®* training is more effective than standard speed training for building muscle strength in beginning exercisers. We therefore recommend this technique as a highly productive strength training protocol. However, *Super Slow®* training is typically characterized as tensive, tedious and tough, so we do not insist on its use. Because we want our participants to be pleased with the exercise process as well as the exercise product, *Super Slow®* training is an optional procedure in our Nautilus facility. However, it has been well-received by our more advanced members, and has produced excellent results for our high-intensity training program participants.

Extending The Exercise Set

Extending the exercise set makes it possible to increase the strength building stimulus by fatiguing more muscle fibers than would normally be used in a standard set of exercise. As illustrated in Figure 7-2, muscle fibers activate and fatigue in a specific order. For example, slow-twitch fibers engage before fast-twitch fibers, but fast-twitch fibers fatigue before slow-twitch fibers. At the end of an exercise set with a given resistance, a certain number of muscle fibers are fatigued. If at this point the resistance is reduced, a few more repetitions may be completed. Although somewhat uncomfortable, this procedure forces more muscle fibers to fatigue and therefore enhances the strength building process.

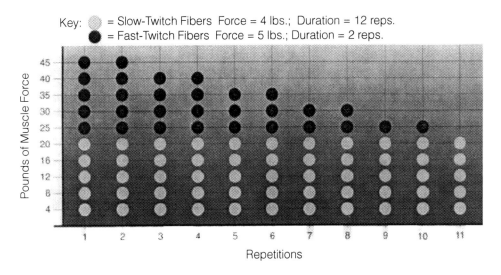

Key: ◯ = Slow-Twitch Fibers Force = 4 lbs.; Duration = 12 reps.
      ● = Fast-Twitch Fibers Force = 5 lbs.; Duration = 2 reps.

Figure 7-2   Hypothetical recruitment and fatigue of slow and fast-twitch muscle fibers during a 10-repetition set of 25-pound triceps extensions.

Two basic procedures for extending the exercise set are known as *breakdown training* and *assisted training.* In breakdown training the participant performs a set of 8 to 12 repetitions to fatigue, then immediately reduces the resistance enough to complete two to five post-fatigue repetitions. We recommend dropping the weightload by about 10 percent for upper body exercises and by about 20 percent for lower body exercises.

In assisted training the exerciser performs a set of 8 to 12 repetitions to fatigue, then receives enough manual assistance from a trainer to complete two to five post-fatigue repetitions. The trainer helps only on the lifting movements (concentric muscle actions) and gives only as much assistance as needed. It is not necessary for the trainer to assist on the lowering movements because our muscles are about 40 percent stronger on eccentric actions. To determine the effectiveness of extended set training we conducted two strength training studies with closely matched beginning exercisers.

Study One: Breakdown Training

In this study, 45 previously sedentary men and women performed one set of 13 Nautilus exercises, three days a week, for eight weeks (Westcott 1997). After four weeks of standard training, half of the subjects performed breakdown training on two of the Nautilus machines (seated leg curl and abdominal). Compared to those who continued standard training, the breakdown training group experienced almost 40 percent greater strength gains (see Figure 7-3).

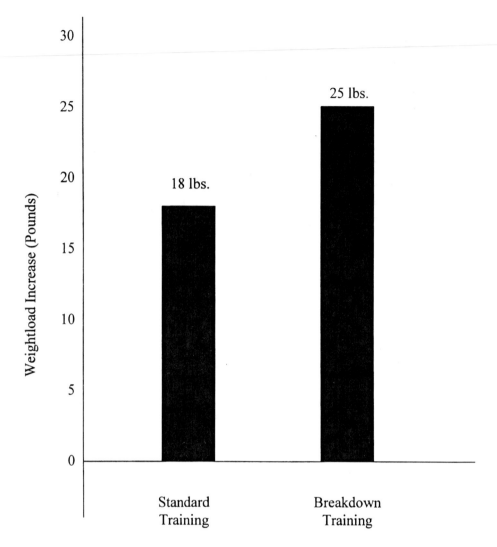

Figure 7-3   Average increase in exercise weightloads after eight weeks of standard or breakdown training with beginner level subjects (45 subjects).

Study Two: Assisted Training

Like the previous study, 42 previously sedentary adults performed one set of 13 Nautilus exercises, three days a week, for eight weeks (Westcott 1997). After four weeks of standard training, half of the subjects performed assisted training on two of the Nautilus machines (seated leg curl and abdominal). Compared to those who continued standard training, the assisted training group experienced 45 percent greater strength gains (see Figure 7-4).

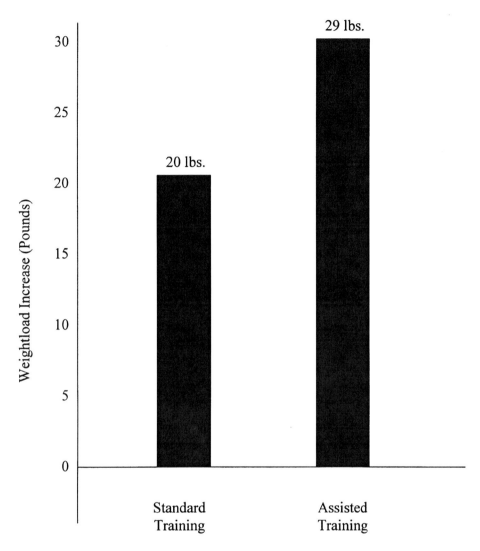

Figure 7-4   Average increase in exercise weightloads after eight weeks of standard or assisted training with beginner level subjects (42 subjects).

The results of these studies indicate that breakdown training and assisted training are more effective than standard training for developing muscle strength in beginning exercisers. We therefore recommend both of these techniques as highly productive strength training protocols. However, due to the discomfort associated with post-fatigue repetitions, we do not require members to train with these methods. Because we want our participants to be pleased with the exercise process as well as the exercise product, breakdown training and assisted training are optional procedures in our Nautilus facility.

Successive Exercises

Another high-intensity technique known as *pre-exhaustion training*, involves two successive exercises for the same muscle group. The first exercise is typically a rotary movement to isolate and fatigue the target muscle. This is followed immediately by a linear movement to further fatigue the target muscle with the help of a fresh assisting muscle. For example, have your client perform 8 to 12 chest crosses to failure to fatigue the pectoralis major muscles. Then move your client as quickly as possible to the bench press and have him or her perform 4 to 6 repetitions to failure to push the pectoralis major muscles to a deeper level of fatigue. This is possible because the bench press exercise uses the fresh triceps muscles as well as the previously worked pectoralis major muscles. After completing both exercises, the pectoralis major muscles should be stressed beyond standard training and experience a greater strength-building stimulus. Our research has shown pre-exhaustion techniques to be highly effective for strength and muscle development (Westcott 1996b).

Of course, the extra effort elicited by the high-intensity training techniques requires more recovery time for muscle remodeling and growth processes. We recommend no more than two high-intensity training sessions per week for best results.

Combined Procedures Program

Our most successful system of high-intensity training is a six-week program that includes all of these exercise techniques. As presented in Table 7-2, the

Week	Exercise Technique	Description
1	Breakdown Training	8-12 reps to failure, then 2-5 reps to failure with 10-20% less resistance.
2	Assisted Training	8-12 reps to failure, then 2-5 reps to failure with manual assistance on lifting phase only.
3	Slow Positive Training	4-6 reps to failure taking 10 seconds for lifting phase and 4 seconds for lowering phase.
4	Slow Negative Training	4-6 reps to failure taking 4 seconds for lifting phase and 10 seconds for lowering phase.
5	Pre-Exhaustion Training	8-12 reps to failure with rotary exercise, then 4-6 reps to failure with linear exercise.
6	Personal Preference	Repeat of favorite high-intensity training technique.

Table 7-2   Six-week program of high-intensity training using all exercise techniques.

participants do one week each of breakdown, assisted, slow positive, slow negative, and pre-exhaustion training, followed by a week of their preferred high-intensity technique. They work all of their major muscle groups in half-hour sessions on Mondays and Fridays with a personal trainer.

As shown in Figure 7-5, a group of 48 advanced exercisers who completed this six-week high-intensity training program made significant improvements in their muscle strength and body composition. Their overall exercise weightloads increased by 17.8 pounds, their lean (muscle) weight increased by 2.5 pounds, and their fat weight decreased by 3.3 pounds. The excellent results achieved by these high-intensity exercisers are particularly impressive considering their relatively brief training sessions (30 minutes each) and low training frequency (two days per week).

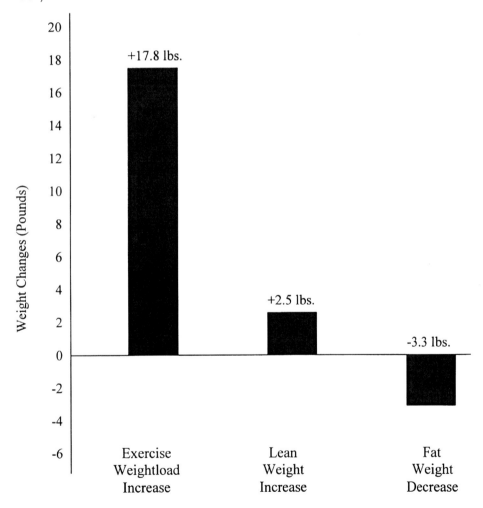

Figure 7-5   Average changes in exercise weightloads and body composition for subjects who performed six weeks of various high-intensity training techniques (48 subjects).

Description Of High-Intensity Training Procedures

There are many methods for incorporating high-intensity training into your clients' strength workouts. However, some of these techniques carry a relatively high risk of injury due to excessive exercise weightloads or training volume, and are therefore not recommended for most practical purposes. The high-intensity procedures that we use include breakdown training, assisted training, slow-positive training, slow-negative training, and pre-exhaustion training. The following section describes each of these techniques, offers training examples, and presents precautions that should be observed for safe, effective and efficient high-intensity workouts. Due to the greater demands imposed by high-intensity training, these techniques should be used in relatively brief and infrequent workouts. Our high-intensity sessions are limited to 30 minutes, two days per week, and we strongly recommend this protocol to prevent overtraining.

Breakdown Training

Breakdown training refers to breaking down the exercise resistance to permit a few additional repetitions after reaching temporary muscle fatigue with the standard weightload. We recommend reducing the resistance just enough to complete two to five post-fatigue repetitions with good form. Generally speaking, this can be accomplished by dropping the weightload by about 10 percent for upper body exercises and about 20 percent for lower body exercises. We advise performing no more than 15 total repetitions per set to keep the training effort within the anaerobic energy system (less than 90 seconds).

Example

Your client performs about 10 repetitions to the point of temporary muscle fatigue with 100 pounds in the seated leg curl exercise. You immediately reduce the weightstack by 20 percent to 80 pounds, and have your client complete as many additional repetitions as possible. If more than five post-fatigue repetitions are completed, reduce the weightload to 85 or 90 pounds next training session, to keep the enhanced exercise set within the anaerobic energy system (90 seconds).

Precautions

Although some highly-motivated individuals may want to do a second breakdown, this is not advisable for most trainees. Double breakdowns are extremely demanding physically and psychologically, and may adversely affect both exercise results and training motivation. One high-effort set of 8 to 12 repetitions followed by two to five good breakdown reps should provide sufficient muscle building stimulus for most clients, and will keep the extended exercise set within the anaerobic energy system (90 seconds).

Assisted Training

Assisted training is similar to breakdown training in that it adds a few extra repetitions at a reduced resistance when the muscle fatigues with the standard weightload. However, there are a couple of differences that may make assisted training even more challenging. Rather than dropping the weightload by a certain amount, the assistant actually helps lift the resistance when the trainee's muscles become too fatigued to do so. That is, you give your client just enough assistance to lift the weightstack two to five more times. Of course, each successive repetition requires more of your assistance due to progressive fatigue in your client's muscles.

Because our muscles are approximately 40 percent stronger in eccentric actions than concentric actions, we can lower about 40 percent more resistance than we can lift. For this reason, you do not give the client assistance on the lowering movements. So, unlike breakdown training in which the weightload is lighter for both the lifting and lowering phases of the post-fatigue repetitions, the resistance is reduced only during performance of the post-fatigue lifting movements. Keep the total number of repetitions to 15 or less to complete the full set within the anaerobic energy system (90 seconds).

Example

Your client performs about 10 repetitions to the point of temporary muscle fatigue with 100 pounds in the leg extension exercise. As he/she attempts a post-fatigue repetition, you provide as much manual assistance as necessary to complete the lifting movement. Allow your client to slowly lower the weightstack without assistance. Repeat this procedure two to five times depending on your client's ability and motivation.

Precautions

The tendency to continue assisted repetitions for more than five post-fatigue repetitions should be avoided, as this training technique requires high muscle effort and can easily be overdone. If appropriate assistance is provided (just enough to complete the lifting movement), two to five additional repetitions should be sufficient and will keep the extended exercise set within the anaerobic energy system (90 seconds).

Slow-Positive Training

The main purpose of slower-speed exercise movements is to reduce the role of momentum and to maximize muscle tension. Slow-positive training is characterized by a 10-second lifting movement and a 4-second lowering movement. We have found that counting 1000-one, 1000-two, and so on, up to 1000-ten is helpful for maintaining a smooth and steady lifting phase. To keep each exercise set within the anaerobic energy system, only four to six repetitions are performed. At 14 seconds per rep, this requires approximately 55 to 85 seconds of continuous muscle tension to complete the training set.

Example

If your client normally does 10 lateral raises with 100 pounds, reduce the resistance by 20 percent to 80 pounds to initiate slow-positive training, This weightload adjustment is advisable to accommodate the loss of momentum and the motor learning associated with the slower movement speed. Have your client perform about five repetitions using the counting technique to facilitate proper exercise form.

Precautions

Due to the longer lifting phase, your clients should not try to exhale throughout the entire concentric muscle action. Instead, they should simply breathe as normally as possible during every repetition. Most important, make sure trainees never hold their breath when performing strength exercise. Remind your clients that although slow speed training is challenging and uncomfortable, each exercise set consists of only four to six repetitions.

Slow-Negative Training

Slow-negative training is similar to slow-positive training, except that the phases are reversed. That is, the lifting phase is performed in four seconds, and the lowering phase is performed in 10 seconds. To keep each exercise set within the anaerobic energy system, only four to six repetitions are performed. At 14 seconds per rep, this requires approximately 55 to 85 seconds of continuous muscle tension to complete the training set. Because eccentric muscle actions are stronger than concentric muscle actions, more resistance can be used in slow-negative training than in slow-positive training. Nonetheless, both techniques minimize momentum and maximize muscle tension resulting in greater strength-building stimulus. We recommend counting 1000-one, 1000-two, and so on, up to 1000-ten, to maintain a smooth and steady lowering phase.

Example

If your client normally performs 10 triceps extensions with 100 pounds, reduce the resistance by 10 percent to 90 pounds for the first slow-negative training session. This weightload adjustment is advisable to accommodate the loss of momentum and the motor learning associated with the slower movement speed. Have your client complete about five repetitions using the counting technique to facilitate proper exercise form.

Precautions

Due to the longer lowering phase, your clients should not attempt to inhale throughout the entire eccentric muscle action. Rather, they should simply breathe as normally as possible during every repetition. Most important, trainees should never hold their breath when performing strength exercise. Remind your clients that although slow speed training is challenging and uncomfortable, each exercise set consists of only four to six repetitions.

Pre-Exhaustion Training

Pre-exhaustion training is essentially successive sets of two exercises for the same target muscle group. For best results, we advise first doing a rotary exercise to isolate and fatigue the target muscle. Follow as quickly as possible with a linear exercise that incorporates a fresh assisting muscle to further fatigue the target muscle. Generally, the first (rotary) exercise should be performed with a resistance that permits about 10 repetitions, and the second (linear) exercise should be performed with a weightload that permits about five repetitions. At a speed of six seconds per repetition, all 15 repetitions will be completed within the anaerobic energy system (90 seconds).

Example

Your client performs about 10 repetitions to the point of temporary muscle fatigue with 100 pounds in the chest cross exercise, which targets the pectoralis major muscles. With as little delay as possible, he/she moves to the bench press machine and performs about five repetitions to the point of temporary muscle fatigue with 150 pounds. The fresh triceps muscles assist the pre-fatigued pectoralis major muscles to complete a few reduced-resistance bench presses, and the two successive chest exercises provide a greater strength stimulus to the pectoralis major muscles.

Precautions

The most important aspect of successful pre-exhaustion training is to transition very quickly between the first (rotary) and second (linear) exercise for the target muscle group. This prevents recovery of the muscle fibers fatigued in the first exercise, and forces other muscle fibers to perform the second exercise. The result is more pervasive muscle fiber fatigue, and a more comprehensive conditioning stimulus that should enhance the muscle-building process. Although some trainees may do a third exercise to reach a deeper level of muscle fatigue, our experience indicates that this may result in overtraining and is therefore not recommended for most participants.

Summary

There are many approaches for overcoming strength plateaus and attaining greater muscle development. However, high-intensity training is undoubtedly the most efficient means for gaining strength and adding muscle. Our recommended high-intensity exercise techniques include breakdown training, assisted training, slow-positive training, slow-negative training, and pre-exhaustion training. Research indicates that these exercise procedures are highly effective for increasing muscle strength and improving body composition.

Our studies with beginning exercisers have shown 40 to 50 percent greater strength gains with breakdown, assisted, and slow-speed training compared to standard training. Our best overall results have been attained from a six-week program involving all of the high-intensity training techniques. Advanced participants who trained just 30 minutes on Mondays and Fridays added 2.5 pounds of lean (muscle) weight and lost 3.3 pounds of fat weight. The positive responses from our high-intensity exercisers clearly support the usefulness of these training techniques and the importance of this program to our fitness participants.

Chapter 8

Heart Start

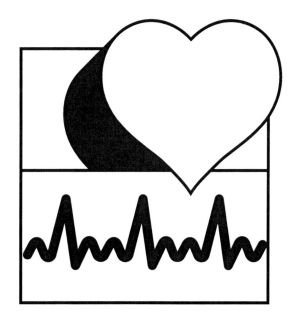

**Heart-Healthy Strength Program
For Cardiac Rehab Patients**

One of the groups that may benefit most from a safe, sensible and supervised program of strength exercise has traditionally avoided this type of activity. These are the men and women who have experienced some degree of cardiovascular disease, such as a heart attack or coronary bypass surgery.

Fortunately, during the past decade many cardiac rehabilitation programs have added strength training to their exercise protocols. Whereas the previous emphasis had been on endurance exercise for cardiovascular conditioning, we now realize that all physical activity affects the heart. We also know that the muscular system and cardiovascular system are interrelated, and that what is beneficial to one is good for both.

For example, most cardiac rehab patients spend considerable time in a hospital bed, and begin their recuperation at a relatively low level of physical fitness. Simple tasks, such as climbing a flight of stairs, may be unusually demanding. However, many of these physical activities are more dependent on muscular strength than cardiovascular endurance. Therefore, the best approach is to combine aerobic conditioning with progressive resistance exercise to make essentially all physical tasks easier to perform. For example, stronger quadriceps, hamstrings and gluteal muscles should reduce the stress of stair climbing and other ambulatory activities. Likewise, stronger upper body muscles should enable cardiac rehab patients to carry groceries, lift grandchildren, and work around the house, yard and garden with less effort.

Research shows that properly performed strength exercise does not adversely affect cardiovascular function, heart rhythm, or blood pressure (Kelemen et al. 1986, Vander et al. 1986, Butler et al. 1987, Stewart et al. 1988, Ghilarducci et al. 1989, Faigenbaum et al. 1990, AACPR 1995, Drought 1995). That is, most cardiac rehab patients can perform appropriate strength training without contraindication, and with confidence that their exercise efforts will enhance their physical fitness and functional ability. To ensure that our program adheres to individual medical guidelines, we require written approval from the patient's physician, as well as any specific recommendations that the doctor desires.

Cardiovascular Response During Strength Exercise

Whenever we perform physical activity our heart rate and systolic blood pressure increase in proportion to the exercise demands. This standard cardiovascular response increases blood flow to the working muscles, supplying oxygen and removing carbon dioxide as necessary.

The American College of Sports Medicine advises that endurance exercise be performed at a level between 60 and 90 percent of maximum heart rate (ACSM 1998). The most common training recommendation is 75 percent of maximum heart rate, which is a safe and comfortable level for most cardiac rehab program participants.

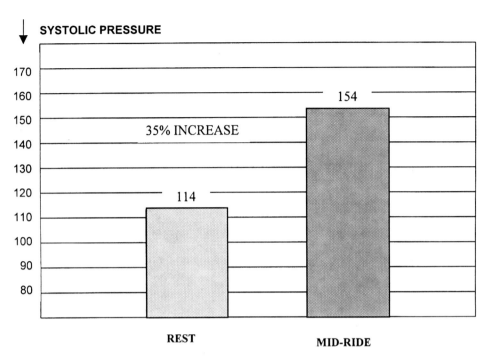

Figure 8-1   Systolic blood pressure response during stationary cycling
(23 subjects)

Steady-state aerobic exercise at 75 percent of maximum heart rate typically raises systolic blood pressure about 35 percent above resting level (Westcott 1991). In other words, if your resting systolic blood pressure is 120 mm Hg, stationary cycling at 75 percent of maximum heart rate will most likely elevate your systolic pressure to about 160 mm Hg and maintain that level throughout the duration of the training session (see Figure 8-1).

Although it has long been assumed that strength training elicits excessive blood pressure responses, this does not appear to be the case when the exercises are performed properly. In fact, upper body strength exercise to the point of muscle fatigue seems to produces a systolic blood pressure response similar to aerobic activity. In one study, subjects performed 10 repetitions to muscle fatigue with about 75 percent of their maximum resistance in the dumbbell curl exercise (Westcott and Howes 1983). Their systolic blood pressure increased progressively with each repetition, reaching about 35 percent above resting level at the point of muscle fatigue (see Figure 8-2 on the next page).

Although working the larger muscles of the lower body results in higher systolic blood pressures, research reveals that these responses are well within safe limits. In a similar study, participants performed 10 repetitions to muscle fatigue on a Nautilus leg press machine (Westcott 1986). Their systolic blood pressure increased progressively repetition-by- repetition, reaching about 50 percent above resting level at the point of muscle fatigue (see Figure 8-3 on the next page).

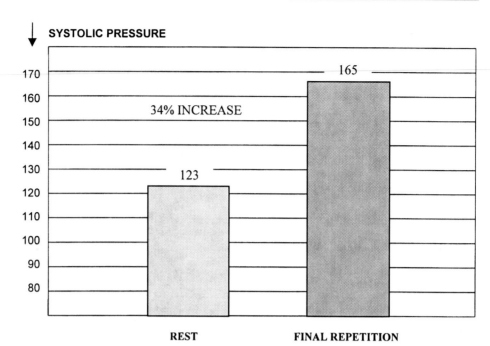

Figure 8-2   Systolic blood pressure response during 10-RM exercise set of one-arm dumbbell curls (24 subjects).

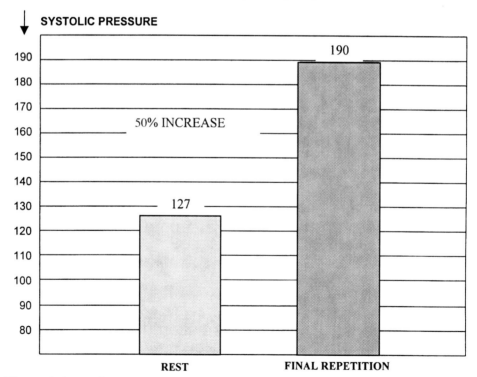

Figure 8-3   Systolic blood pressure response during 10-RM exercise set of Nautilus leg presses (25 subjects).

In this study, the subjects' resting systolic blood pressure averaged 127 mm Hg, and their peak exercise systolic blood pressure averaged 190 mm Hg. While higher than the upper body blood pressure response to resistance exercise, this systolic blood pressure level is far below the American College of Sports Medicine exercise guideline of 225 mm Hg.

Following the final repetition, systolic blood pressure drops quickly towards resting level. In fact, as presented in Figure 8.4, a study with 100 men and women of all ages showed a return to resting blood pressure readings within one minute of completing an 11-machine Nautilus circuit (Westcott and Pappas 1987).

The findings from these studies suggest that properly performed strength training does not elicit excessive or dangerous blood pressure responses. While proper exercise performance includes a variety of technical considerations, the two major factors are continuous breathing and continuous movement. That is, exercisers should exhale during lifting movements, inhale during lowering movements, and *never* hold their breath. Breath-holding while performing resistance exercise can produce seriously high blood pressure responses. Likewise, exercisers should *not* hold the resistance in a static position for more than a moment, as isometric muscle contractions can also cause seriously elevated blood pressures.

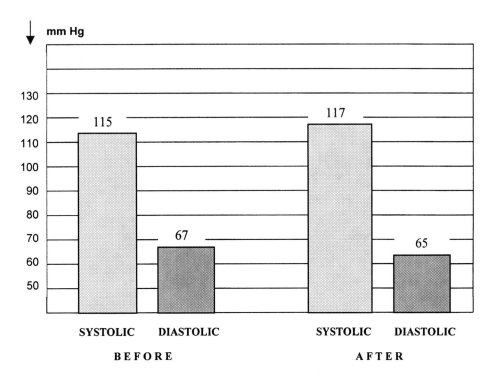

Figure 8-4 Blood pressure readings sixty seconds before and after performing an eleven-station Nautilus circuit strength training session (100 subjects).

Heart Rate Monitoring

While it is not very practical to monitor your clients' blood pressure when they are performing strength exercise, you can easily take their heart rate while they train. Fortunately, heart rate and systolic blood pressure follow a similar response pattern during a set of strength exercise. Both increase progressively as additional repetitions are completed.

We recently conducted research on the heart rate response to strength training at two levels of resistance (Westcott and O'Grady 1998). All of the subjects performed the following Nautilus exercises to the point of muscle fatigue with both 70 and 85 percent of their maximum resistance: leg extension, leg curl, bench press, biceps curl. On average, they completed almost 14 repetitions to fatigue with 70 percent of maximum resistance, and just over 7 repetitions to fatigue with 85 percent of maximum resistance. Interestingly, each resistance level resulted in essentially the same heart rate elevation, namely 123 beats per minute. This represented about 50 beats above the subjects' resting heart rate and just under 70 percent of their predicted maximum heart rate.

Although both resistance levels produced similar end points with respect to heart rate, the increase per repetition was considerably greater when using the heavier weightloads. With 70 percent of maximum resistance, the subjects' heart rate increased about four beats per repetition. However, when using 85 percent of maximum resistance, the subjects' heart rate increased almost seven beats per repetition. Consequently, training with 70 percent of maximum resistance may be preferable from a cardiovascular perspective, as it offers more heart rate control on a repetition-by-repetition basis. Table 8-1 presents specific information on the average exercise repetitions and heart rate responses when training with these two resistance levels.

	Mean Repetitions Completed (Reps)	Mean Peak Heart Rate (Beats/Min)	Mean Percentage of Maximum Heart Rate (Percent)	Mean Heart Rate Increase Over Resting (Beats/Min)	Mean Heart Rate Increase Per Repetition (Beats/Min)
70 Percent Maximum Resistance	13.5	123	69	53	3.9
85 Percent Maximum Resistance	7.6	122	68	52	6.5

Table 8-1 Repetitions and heart rate responses to strength training with 70 and 85 percent of maximum resistance (25 subjects).

Heart Rate Guidelines

As illustrated in Figure 8-5, heart rate increases progressively and predictably during a set of strength exercise to muscle fatigue with both 70 and 85 percent of maximum resistance. Because heart rate increases more gradually when training with 70 rather than 85 percent of maximum resistance, we consider the lower weightload more conservative and therefore more desirable for post-coronary participants.

Consider a cardiac rehab patient who wants to develop muscle strength but is not to exceed 50 percent of his maximum heart rate during exercise. After an introductory period using relatively light weights and low effort, we suggest progressing to 70 percent of maximum resistance. As indicated on the heart rate/ repetition graph, his heart rate should reach 50 percent of maximum at about 10 repetitions (see Figure 8-5). He would therefore train with 70 percent of maximum resistance to stimulate strength development, but he would perform only 10

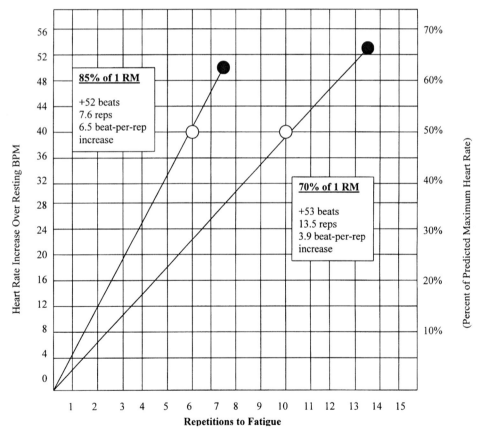

Figure 8-5   Mean reps to fatigue and mean heart rate increase at 70% and 85% of maximum resistance.
○ indicates number of reps performed at 40 heart beats above resting level or at 50% of maximum heart rate.

repetitions with this resistance to keep his heart rate below 50 percent of maximum heart rate.

The heart rate response to performing repetitions with 70 percent of maximum resistance is linear, increasing about four beats per repetition. Therefore, it is relatively easy to design an appropriate training protocol for the desired heart rate. For example, performing eight repetitions with 70 percent of maximum resistance should raise his exercise heart rate to about 40 percent of maximum heart rate (see Figure 8-5).

Unfortunately, this relationship loses accuracy at lower repetition ranges. For this reason, Figure 8.5 also presents the heart beats over resting level for progressive repetitions with 70 percent of maximum resistance. For example, performing 8 repetitions with 70 percent of maximum resistance increases heart rate approximately 32 beats above resting level, and completing 10 repetitions raises heart rate about 40 beats above resting level. So, if a physician wants a client to stay within 40 beats of resting heart rate, a training protocol of 10 repetitions with 70 percent of maximum resistance should be appropriate.

Sample Strength Training Program

There are numerous examples of safe and successful strength training programs for post-coronary patients. In general, however, it makes sense to start slowly, introducing just two resistance exercises per week with clear instruction, careful supervision and continuous heart rate monitoring. Let's assume that Kim has successfully completed a hospital-based cardiac rehabilitation program, and she wants to continue her exercise program in a supervised setting. Her cardiologist recommends 20 to 30 minutes of treadmill walking or stationary cycling, and up to 12 basic strength exercises for the major muscle groups, three days per week. Kim's training heart rate is not to exceed 40 beats above her resting level of 70 beats per minute.

We recommend that Kim wear a heart rate monitor every training session, during both her aerobic activity and strength exercise. We also suggest that Kim begin her workouts with about 10 minutes of walking, then perform her strength exercises, and finish with about 10 minutes of stationary cycling. If she has not previously done strength training, two resistance exercises should be sufficient for the first week. Thereafter we advise adding two strength exercises a week as presented in Table 8-2. Kim could also increase her walking and cycling durations by one minute each on successive weeks, until she totals 20 minutes of endurance exercise at a heart rate below 110 beats per minute.

During the first couple of weeks, the strength exercise weightloads should be relatively light to maintain Kim's heart rate around 95 beats per minute. As she becomes more competent and confident with her strength workouts, the resistance can be increased to attain heart rates near 110 beats per minute as indicated in Table 8.2. The 110 heart rate should be achieved by performing 10 controlled

Week	Nautilus Exercise	Target Muscles	Sets	Reps	Peak Heart Rate
1	Bench Press	Pectoralis Major Triceps	1	5	90 bpm
	Compound Row	Latissimus Dorsi Biceps	1	5	90 bpm
2	Leg Press	Quadriceps Hamstrings	1	6	94 bpm
	Bench Press	Pectoralis Major Triceps	1	6	94 bpm
	Compound Row	Latissimus Dorsi Biceps	1	6	94 bpm
	Lateral Raise	Deltoids	1	6	94 bpm
3	Leg Press	Quadriceps Hamstrings	1	7	98 bpm
	Bench Press	Pectoralis Major Triceps	1	7	98 bpm
	Compound Row	Latissimus Dorsi Biceps	1	7	98 bpm
	Lateral Raise	Deltoids	1	7	98 bpm
	Low Back	Erector Spinae	1	7	98 bpm
	Abdominal	Rectus Abdominis	1	7	98 bpm
4	Leg Press	Quadriceps Hamstrings	1	8	102 bpm
	Bench Press	Pectoralis Major Triceps	1	8	102 bpm
	Compound Row	Latissimus Dorsi Biceps	1	8	102 bpm
	Lateral Raise	Deltoids	1	8	102 bpm
	Biceps Curl	Biceps	1	8	102 bpm
	Triceps Extension	Triceps	1	8	102 bpm
	Low Back	Erector Spinae	1	8	102 bpm
	Abdominal	Rectus Abdominis	1	8	102 bpm
5	Leg Press	Quadriceps Hamstrings	1	9	106 bpm
	Leg Curl	Hamstrings	1	9	106 bpm
	Leg Extension	Quadriceps	1	9	106 bpm
	Bench Press	Pectoralis Major Triceps	1	9	106 bpm
	Compound Row	Latissimus Dorsi Biceps	1	9	106 bpm

Continued

Week	Nautilus Exercise	Target Muscles	Sets	Reps	Peak Heart Rate
5	Lateral Raise	Deltoids	1	9	106 bpm
(cont.)	Biceps Curl	Biceps	1	9	106 bpm
	Triceps Extension	Triceps	1	9	106 bpm
	Low Back	Erector Spinae	1	9	106 bpm
	Abdominal	Rectus Abdominis	1	9	106 bpm
6	Leg Press	Quadriceps Hamstrings	1	10	110 bpm
	Leg Curl	Hamstrings	1	10	110 bpm
	Leg Extension	Quadriceps	1	10	110 bpm
	Hip Adduction	Hip Adductors	1	10	110 bpm
	Hip Abduction	Hip Abductors	1	10	110 bpm
	Bench Press	Pectoralis Major Triceps	1	10	110 bpm
	Compound Row	Latissimus Dorsi Biceps	1	10	110 bpm
	Lateral Raise	Deltoids	1	10	110 bpm
	Biceps Curl	Biceps	1	10	110 bpm
	Triceps Extension	Triceps	1	10	110 bpm
	Low Back	Erector Spinae	1	10	110 bpm
	Abdominal	Rectus Abdominis	1	10	110 bpm
7	Same as Week 6 with slightly higher resistance as necessary to attain heart rate of 110 bpm.				
8	Same as Week 7 with slightly higher resistance as necessary to attain heart rate of 110 bpm.				

After two months of strength training, it is suggested that the patient be re-evaluated by his or her cardiologist, and that the training intensity be adjusted accordingly.

Table 8-2   Sample progressive strength training program for post-coronary patients based on 70 percent of maximum resistance. As strength increases, weightloads must also be increased proportionately. Use peak heart rate response as the criteria for adding resistance. Resting heart rate assumed to be 70 beats per minute.

repetitions with 70 percent of maximum resistance, as this resistance typically produces a heart rate increase of about four beats per repetition (10 reps x 4 bpm = 40 bpm). When 10 repetitions no longer elicit 110 beats per minute, Kim can perform more repetitions with the same weightload or increase the resistance by one to three pounds.

If everything goes according to plan, Kim should make excellent progress, improve her physical fitness and develop a higher functional capacity. Assuming that this occurs, Kim's cardiologist may allow her to train at a higher intensity and establish a new exercise heart rate level, such as 50 beats above resting (120 beats per minute). In this case, Kim may either do additional repetitions with her present weightload (70 percent maximum), or raise the resistance (75 to 85 percent of maximum) for more strength- building benefit.

Summary

Research shows that most post-coronary patients respond positively to sensible and supervised strength training, and that properly performed resistance exercise does not adversely affect cardiovascular function, heart rhythm or blood pressure. Studies demonstrated similar heart rate and blood pressure responses to endurance exercise and strength exercise, both of which enhance patients' physical fitness and functional ability. Strength training with 70 percent of maximum resistance to muscle fatigue raises heart rate about 50 beats per minute above resting level, and elevates systolic blood pressure up to 50 percent above resting level. Both increases are well within normal exercise ranges. Heart rate increases about four beats per repetition when training with 70 percent of maximum resistance, which makes it possible to control heart rate elevation by the number of repetitions performed with this weightload.

Chapter 9

Workout on Wheels

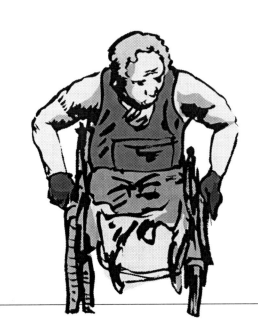

Upper Body Strength Program
for Wheelchair Users

Every year approximately 7,800 individuals experience spinal cord injuries (SCI) and join the estimated 250,000 to 400,000 Americans living with either a spinal cord injury or serious spinal dysfunction. Majorities of these people are males between the ages of 16-30, whose injuries occur following motor vehicle accidents (42%), acts of violence (24%), falls (22%), and sporting accidents (8%) (Miller 1995, NSCIA 1999). Diseases such as polio, spina bifida, and multiple sclerosis also cause damage to the spinal cord that may result in partial paralysis and the need for a wheelchair. Training principles and techniques represented in this chapter will primarily focus on the needs of individuals whose paralysis is the result of injury.

For SCI individuals, better fitness levels may mean a higher quality of life by more easily accomplishing daily tasks such as transferring from a wheelchair, jumping a curb, reaching for objects, or wheeling for extended distances. Better fitness is also useful for developing greater skill and challenge in sports such as scuba diving, bi- or mono-skiing, marathoning, sled hockey, swimming, wheelchair rugby, basketball, tennis and archery. Exercise may also help prevent some complications commonly associated with this type of injury or illness such as cardiovascular disease and diabetes. Muscle conditioning through strength exercise may help reduce muscle atrophy and bone degeneration caused by disuse (Kaplan et al. 1981, Gross et al. 1997). Strength training may also increase the individual's resting metabolism and counter the inevitable obesity that results from immobility and muscle loss. Finally, it can provide important psychological and social benefits (Schack 1991, Schulz and Decker 1985). Muscle conditioning and cardiovascular endurance are imperative for the person who *works out on wheels*.

By establishing a program largely operated by well-trained volunteer fitness assistants, the South Shore YMCA provides a low-cost, time-efficient, and highly productive strength exercise program for those who are unable to train independently. For the past ten years, student interns, members of our fitness center, members of the community, personal care attendants, and many of our fitness staff have generously given of their time to team up with disabled partners. Unsolicited comments by our members reveal the inspiration they receive by witnessing the dedication and character of the individuals in our Partnership Program. Frequent conversations with YMCA members, participants, and staff indicate overwhelmingly that expansion of services to the disabled enhances the quality of our organization by providing a valuable personal experience for all. Relationships spring up naturally among able-bodied and disabled members who share common experiences, humor, and mutual respect. Often, simply observing the Partnership Program in process shatters glass walls of ignorance regarding fitness for the disabled.

Our participants appreciate the opportunity to mainstream into a healthy, nonmedical fitness environment that doubles as a social setting. For many people who have suffered injury, the fitness center is the first place outside of hospital, friends, and family where SCI individuals test their abilities and acceptance.

Supportive social ties are very important to disabled participants. In fact, research indicates that such connections play a significant role in the survival and longevity of these individuals (Trieschmann 1988).

Non-disabled members welcome SCI members readily and feel good about an organization that recognizes everyone's need and ability to work toward better health and fitness. Both able-bodied and disabled members are encouraged by the discipline and commitment demonstrated every day by our Partnership Program members and their trainers.

Setting Up A Program

Getting the Word Out

You may wish to begin your program for people with disabilities on a small scale, as we did, with a few SCI members training one-on-one in your main facility during low-use times under the supervision of an on-duty fitness instructor. This keeps program costs to a minimum, and allows your staff to oversee the main facility while simultaneously working with participants.

As the program grows, or if you begin to experience increased membership in your center, these demands may restrict your ability to use paid staff to provide constant one-on-one service. You will need a system of staff recruitment that continues to keep participant costs to a minimum while maintaining one-on-one training. When our own fitness center exploded with new memberships, we decided to train student interns and adaptive fitness class members from various colleges and universities who wished to include this exercise experience in their education. We also recruited volunteers. These individuals were usually sought in-house by posting signs in our Nautilus Center and other areas of the Y, or advertising in our YMCA or Partnership Program newsletters. We found that many respondents were interested in getting involved because they regularly saw the program in action while they performed their own fitness training in our facility.

When we were able to accommodate more program participants, they were recruited by sending flyers and informational letters to local physical therapy centers and hospitals specializing in SCI. Information was mailed to the Center for Information on Disabilities, as well as to nearby universities with student centers for the disabled. Word of mouth proved to be an excellent referral method. Participants often discussed our program with friends and acquaintances, and motivated them to get involved. As we contacted healthcare professionals for medical referrals and consultations, they became excited about the program and requested flyers for other patients (Ramsden 1994).

Program Protocol

Over the years our program has served numerous SCI individuals, as well as people with various other disabilities. We have found that our protocols for intake, volunteer staff training, and exercise-training regimens work very well to maintain high standards of safety and service.

Reasonable Accommodations

Our fitness center is fully accessible according to the Americans with Disabilities Act (ADA) requirements. However, when appropriate, we arrange any additional reasonable accommodations such as having someone available to open nonelectronic doors. In most cases the volunteer trainer meets the participant in our Snack Bar area, which is fully accessible by means of electronic entrances.

Unless SCI individuals wish to exercise in our swimming pool, most choose not to use the locker rooms, although these are readily available. In addition to the locker facilities, we offer two separate changing rooms that allow privacy for assistance by a family member, personal care attendant, or friend. Our staff does not assist with these personal care services.

Rest rooms are accessible and nearby our training center. Our staff do not usually need to assist with this service, since most wheelchair participants have relieved their bladder directly before arriving at our center, and/or are relatively independent. In the event of an emergency, however, a staff person should be available for assistance.

Transportation

Participants are required to provide their own transportation to our site. Many are able to drive, including some high-level quadriplegic participants who have fully-adaptable vans. Others have family members or friends who are able to provide this service. When requested, we refer people without transportation to a local agency that provides van service by appointment for a small fee.

The Initial Contact

The Partnership Program Director is the primary contact person when an individual calls the Y to inquire about our program. It is helpful if the Program Director has a degree in physical therapy, or education in the area of adaptive fitness, and experience working with the disabled in an exercise arena. The director takes information from the prospective member regarding the nature and level of disability, and the special needs of the individual. The director also records the person's address and telephone number, a family member's telephone number, and numbers of the physical therapist, occupational therapist, personal care attendant, and/or physician treating the individual. Days and hours of availability, and areas of exercise interest such as strength training, cardiovascular exercise, and swimming are also recorded.

We often do an initial telephone consult with a physical therapist, or in some cases, with the participant's personal physician to confirm that our training regimen is appropriate for the unique needs of the individual. Information regarding our exercise equipment and procedures may be sent to the medical professional. In most cases we receive a positive recommendation for the individual to participate in the program. In all cases we adhere to guidelines or restrictions given by the physicians and therapists. Sometimes a physical therapist will visit our site during the first training session for input and observation. Usually, medical professionals are happy to assist us in establishing a fitness program. They know that the health benefits to their patients are well worth their efforts, and that physical therapy services do not provide lifelong exercise programming. They appreciate a fitness center that takes a proactive role in health and fitness *for all*.

The Personal Consultation

It is always important to meet with candidates prior to acceptance into the program:

1. to ensure that we can serve the individual's needs based on the extent of his or her illness or injury.
2. to acclimate him or her to our staff and facilities.
3. to go over any accessibility concerns.
4. to answer questions regarding logistics, such as the location of rest rooms, water fountains, and the parking area.
5. to help him or her feel comfortable and confident in our fitness center.
6. to fill out a program application.
7. to fill out a medical history form.

Medical History Questionnaires

As with all new YMCA members, we require each participant to fill out a medical history questionnaire (refer to Appendix C). For Partnership Program members, this is usually done at the initial interview. Although similar to the form for non-disabled members, we add specific questions for disabled participants to help instructors determine such things as the level of injury to the spine, the date of injury, whether the participant has difficulty breathing, blood pressure concerns, and other symptoms that may affect training. The level of injury will determine how much training assistance the volunteer instructor will need to provide. The date of injury may indicate whether the participant has been sedentary for an extended period of time, has newly recovered from an injury, has recently completed a physical therapy program, and/or is psychologically adjusting to the implications of the injury.

A number of questions also address conditions commonly associated with SCI. These will be discussed in detail in a later section of this chapter. Finally, as on all medical history questionnaires, we ask whether the participant has consulted with his or her physician prior to joining the program. In most cases we contact the physician or physical therapist directly to discuss our program in greater detail.

Training The Trainers

Many Partnership Program volunteer trainers have had previous experience in strength training due to their educational background and/or personal experience. However, each new volunteer trainer undergoes a minimum of three sessions of one-on-one, hands-on training with a Master Trainer in order to become familiar with the specialized equipment and the exercise protocol. The Master Trainer is a staff person with advanced knowledge and experience providing exercise to disabled individuals, and is able to alert the volunteer trainer about contraindications to exercise, and special considerations when training a new participant. It is especially helpful if the Master Trainer is a physical therapist experienced in working with spinal cord injuries.

The Master Trainer initially trains the new staff volunteer on the equipment as if the volunteer *is* the SCI participant. This allows the new staff member to understand on some level what the experience might be like for a first-time member coming to our center with a disability. The second session reviews basic exercise instruction covered in session one. It also includes how to secure the wheelchair, and allows the volunteer to gain experience by training the Master Trainer as if he or she were the participant. In this manner, the Master Trainer is able to provide positive feedback, offer suggestions, give encouragement, and address any training questions. During the third session the new staff person practices training the Master Trainer again and goes through a final review.

When the Master Trainer is confident that the volunteer is well-prepared, the first exercise session with the SCI member is arranged. The Master Trainer always attends the first session to provide support and any additional instruction or supervision that may not have been anticipated. The Master Trainer continues to be present at the exercise sessions until the fitness routine is performed well by both partners, and until the volunteer demonstrates full confidence in training without additional supervision. Usually this takes no more than one or two sessions to accomplish.

Keeping Participants Motivated

Motivation for the SCI individual comes in various forms. Many of our participants were previously athletes and therefore already appreciate the challenge of driving one's self to new heights of accomplishment. Some of our SCI members are motivated to obtain greater life skills by developing a stronger body. Others participate in various sports and recreational activities, and find strength training useful in raising their performance level.

Knowledgeable instructors share their expertise continuously and vary the training protocol to help participants stay excited about their fitness program. Providing educational materials on exercise benefits and proper technique also generates fitness enthusiasm. Training seminars for participants and staff on adaptive fitness topics such as wheelchair transfers, developing inclusive group exercise programs, and making the fitness center more adaptable are very popular at our facility. Listening to the ideas of program participants is also important. Offering special activities such as wheelchair basketball for mixed groups of able-bodied and disabled participants is an enjoyable way to get many people involved in sports interaction. Finally, the atmosphere created by caring staff and friendly members can make a major difference in encouraging disabled individuals to give the exercise program a try.

Exercise Protocol

Overview of the Equipment

Fitness programs can be adapted on either Nautilus machines or specially-designed equipment for wheelchair accessibility such as the Bow Flex VersaTrainer. Equipment selection depends on the extent of the injury and the ability of the participant to grip machine handles and transfer in and out of the wheelchair. Wrist cuffs and some designs of weight training gloves may also help determine which equipment you and your client wish to use.

Although our VersaTrainer is designed specifically for wheelchair use, most members with paraplegia prefer the Nautilus equipment, as they are able to transfer onto many machines easily and can perform the exercises with little or no assistance. Quadriplegic individuals, who comprise the majority of our Partnership Program wheelchair participants, require the assistance of a training partner and do most of their exercises from the wheelchair on a VersaTrainer or other wheelchair-accessible apparatus.

Some of these exercisers are also able to transfer onto selected Nautilus machines, with assistance from our staff. *If a fitness trainer is uncertain about his or her participant's capabilities, frank discussion is necessary for safety purposes, and is always appreciated by the individual being trained.* Fitness trainers who are uncomfortable helping transfer participants onto the machines, or who have physical limitations restricting their ability to do so, should not be matched with clients who wish to transfer onto the equipment. As with any of your members, safety is of maximum importance. Staff should be fully trained in assisting with wheelchair transfers if they are to be helping in this capacity. It is best to have an additional fitness instructor available to help with the transfer. For everyone's benefit, staff and volunteers should be encouraged to express any concerns or hesitations regarding their respective training situations, and should only assist with this program if they feel fully comfortable with their responsibilities.

Physical Considerations When Developing A Fitness Program For SCI Members

It is important to understand that being disabled does not necessarily mean being "*unabled.*" Perhaps a better term would be "differently-abled," or doing things in a way that is most suitable to the unique requirements of the individual at hand.

In actuality, this concept applies equally to able-bodied and disabled clients, since most fitness participants have various physical conditions and/or considerations that factor into the design of their training program.

In order to best serve the needs of our SCI members, and to ensure the safety and productivity of a training regimen, it is necessary for your staff to understand the nature of the SCI condition, and the physical complications often associated with this illness or injury. Awareness of these factors usually helps trainers become more confident and competent working with SCI individuals. Guidance by Master Trainers during the participant's initial training sessions is essential.

The Physiology of an SCI Injury

The *spinal column* is the series of vertebrae that enclose the spinal cord and form the backbone. The *spinal cord* is the network of the central nervous system that extends from the brain through the spinal canal. In a healthy individual the spinal cord delivers instructions from the brain to various muscles of the body indicating whether to contract or relax.

Damage to the spinal cord causes a loss of functional mobility, a loss of sensation—or sometimes both—to the area at or below the point of injury. It is important to note that although upon initial injury a muscle may no longer function as a result of SCI, the muscle itself has not been damaged (Miller 1995). Rather, it is the disruption of the *connecting nerves* that leads to partial or complete paralysis.

This is sometimes compared to telephone wires downed in a storm. The telephones themselves are perfectly operational, but the damaged wires leading to the phones prevent proper function. So also, for a person with SCI, the brain and muscles remain in tact, but cannot be connected to each other due to *damaged wiring.* The same principle is true for the loss of *feeling* that occurs in an affected area. Partial or complete loss of sensation results when damage occurs to the connection of nerve to the skin and joint receptors (Miller 1995).

Common Medical Conditions Resulting From SCI

Individuals with SCI may develop other medical conditions as a result of their injury. Urinary tract infections and respiratory complications are common. Loss of healthy nerve connections to the bladder or bowels sometimes leads to incontinence. When establishing a training program for someone with incontinence it may be helpful to gently suggest relieving his or her bladder prior to exercise, as this activity can stimulate the need to urinate. This may also prevent the onset of autonomic dysreflexia, which is sometimes brought on by a full bladder.

Autonomic dysreflexia is a condition signaled by a pounding headache, sweating forehead, goose bumps, and/or a stuffy nose. Blood pressure elevates rapidly to dangerously high levels, and can result in cerebral hemorrhage if it is not treated as a medical emergency. To help prevent this condition, ask your participant to use the rest room prior to your training session, or just before leaving the house to come to the fitness center (Trieschmann 1988).

Within the first five years of a spinal cord injury, 25-30% of individuals will be hospitalized with pressure sores (Trieschmann 1988). These are caused by poor circulation and skin breakdown in weight bearing areas, and can develop into serious and sometimes life-threatening conditions if not treated (Miller 1995). Pressure sores occur primarily in the buttocks and sacral area, the heels, ankles and hips (Trieschmann 1988). Usually SCI individuals are carefully monitored by health care professionals for these problems, and prompt care is given.

Sometimes situations such as these may require an adaptation in training, may result in absenteeism from the fitness center, or occasionally necessitate the hospitalization of your clients. If there is going to be an extended absence of a few weeks or so, it is helpful to let participants know that when health considerations are resolved, their training partners will be ready to promptly return to exercise. Otherwise, it may be assumed that training partners will be assigned to other individuals, and your participants may become discouraged, particularly if there is a waiting list for the program. When your clients are able to return, be sure to lower the training weightloads accordingly and progress gradually.

If for any reason a participant is not able to return to the program for several months, it may be best to allow the trainer to work with a new client. When the SCI member is ready to resume an exercise program, immediately place them at the top of the list for a fitness partner, as continuity of training is important.

Physical Considerations During Exercise

Several factors are important in deciding how to properly train your participant. Determining your client's motor control or coordination, balance and trunk stability, spasticity, range of motion, pain, muscle function, sensation, and fatigue levels prior to the start of training will help you understand better how to proceed (Miller 1995). You will also gain information by asking your client the level of injury to the spine.

A complete injury refers to maximum damage to the spinal cord at the point of injury, resulting in entire paralysis and loss of sensation at the point of injury and below, equally affecting both the left and right sides of the body. An incomplete injury refers to partial damage to the spinal cord, resulting in some dysfunction and/ or loss of sensation and movement at the point of injury and below. Left and right sides of the body may vary in effects of the injury (Spinal Cord Injury 1999). See Table 9-1 for general guidelines on affected areas depending on the site of the injury. No two injuries are exactly alike, however, and your client will be able to provide you with information specific to his or her abilities. If there are questions as to appropriate exercise protocol, consult with the individual's physician or physical therapist directly, especially regarding conditions such as spasticity, joint contractures, and/or tenodesis.

Spasticity results from muscle and tendon imbalances caused by the injury. Evidenced by uncontrolled and exaggerated movement of the limbs, spasticity is best controlled by slow movement speed when strength training. Stretch reflexes

There are 8 cervical vertebrae in the neck. (C)
There are 12 thoracic vertebrae in the chest area. (T)
There are 5 lumbar vertebrae in the lower back. (L)
There are 5 sacral vertebrae in the pelvic area. (S)

Injury Level	Functional Capacity
C1 & C2	No motor function below the chin. Unable to breathe without a respirator.
C3	Paralysis below neck. Possibly some shoulder function. May breathe with respirator.
C4	Independent breathing. Upper extremities paralyzed.
C5	Use of shoulders and biceps. Some upper arm mobility.
C6	May be able to transfer from wheelchair. Wrist control. No finger function. Use thumb crotch and index finger.
C7	Independent, but finger dexterity impaired for some use of hands.
T1 – T8	Paraplegia, control of the hands, fairly good breathing ability. Poor trunk control.
T9 – T12	Good abdominal control, excellent seated balance & trunk stability.
L1 – L5	Decreasing control of hip flexors and legs.
S1 – S5	Decreasing control of hip flexors and legs.
Sources:	Trieschmann, Roberta B., Ph.D. (1988) Spinal Cord Injuries: Psychological, Social, and Vocational Rehabilitation, 2nd Edition. Demos Publications, New York , New York.
	Spinal Cord Injury: Spinal Cord 101, Basic Anatomy, **www.spinalinjury.net**.

Table 9-1   Levels of injury to the spine and corresponding functional capacity.

may actually trigger the onset of spastic movements, and therefore prolonged static stretching or relaxation may be the best techniques to use. If your client demonstrates an increase in spasticity or a decrease in function during or following exercise, modify or stop the training. When uncertain, contact the participant's physical therapist or physician to determine how to proceed.

Certain conditions, including spasticity, can sometimes lead to joint contractures, which shorten muscle and connective tissue and reduce range of motion in the affected joint. Some types of contractures are temporary, while others are permanent. If your client has a reduced range of joint movement you should discuss this with his or her physical therapist prior to beginning your training program. If single joint movements cannot be isolated during exercise, then your client should probably not perform strength exercise. You should also not force joint range of motion (Miller 1995).

Flexibility training, in many instances is beneficial for the exerciser. However, there are certain times when it is best to allow limbs to remain tight for functional purposes. Tenodesis is a condition whereby the SCI participant is unable to release the affected hand from a gripping position. This may actually be helpful to your client, since paralysis prevents movement, and since keeping the hand in the cupped position allows the participant to perform various day-to-day functions that would otherwise be impossible (Miller 1995). Gradually stretching the hand to an opened position may limit the participant's ability to use the hand productively. This is another instance where the physical therapist will know what is best for your client.

Autonomic Nervous System Impairment

The autonomic nervous system (ANS) regulates several physiological functions. In a non-disabled individual this system works to ensure that the body is able to meet the demands of exercise and adjust itself to the increased load of activity. In disabled individuals the ANS may have become impaired, particularly if the injury is at a T1 – T5 level or higher. With regard to exercise, you may see the following (Miller 1995):

- reduced aerobic and muscular exercise capacity
- inability of the heart rate to reach a level higher than 120 beats per minute
- slower blood pressure responses to exercise
- impaired blood circulation
- fatigue
- impaired sweating
- cold or heat sensitivity

It is best to begin training your SCI participant with a very light weight setting, increasing repetitions only as tolerated, and increasing weightloads gradually. Besides being best for your client's reduced aerobic and muscular exercise capacity, this milder form of training may also help prevent complications from the other impairments listed above.

Temperature regulation problems may cause your client to have an inability to shiver and conserve heat in cold weather. Conversely, in warm climates your participant may not be able to perspire and dissipate heat. In the case of cold sensitivity, try adding layers of clothing to keep the member warm while training.

If your client is sensitive to heat, have the participant wear lightweight clothing and train in an air-conditioned environment. To counteract impaired sweating, use a spray bottle or damp towel to cool down the participant periodically, and be sure to provide adequate hydration.

Additional Staff Training and Education

Besides educating the exercise instructors in your program for people with disabilities, all fitness staff should be aware of how to interact on at least a minimum level with special needs individuals. Whether a person is blind or deaf, has multiple sclerosis, spina bifida, cerebral palsy, developmental disabilities, mental retardation, or some other challenging condition, you are almost certain to receive inquiries at some time about training these individuals in your fitness center. Your staff should know how to provide reasonable accommodations, or have a contact person they can refer to when someone with unique physical requirements joins your facility.

You may want to invite an adaptive exercise consultant to do a workshop series for interested staff on topics such as proper wheelchair transfer techniques, dehydration and rehydration, adapting movements for people with physical disabilities, and/or fitness programming for this population. If you wish, the educational series can be designed to incorporate disabilities other than SCI injury, including potentially progressive diseases such as multiple sclerosis, muscular dystrophy, and post-polio syndrome. It can also include exercise communication techniques for the deaf and blind. Contact the hospital or physical therapy center nearest you that treats spinal cord injuries or other disabilities and ask if they can recommend a consultant. A university in your area that offers an exercise science curriculum may also have a faculty member specializing in adaptive fitness who is available for presentations. The Center for Information on Disabilities may also be a good resource.

For more comprehensive staff training, the American Council on Exercise (ACE) offers a *Clinical Exercise Specialist Certification*, which prepares fitness professionals for working with people who are disabled, undergoing rehabilitation, or experiencing chronic illness. You may reach ACE at (800) 825-3636, or view their website at www.acefitness.org. In this specialized field of training there is always more to learn.

There are also some excellent books on fitness training for people with disabilities. One such book, which has been referred to extensively in this chapter is *Fitness Programming and Physical Disability,* edited by Patricia D. Miller. You will find in-depth chapters by notable experts on many topics we have included here, and more.

As you glean information from various sources you may want to develop a notebook of relevant information for your staff to review. Keep the notebook in the training facility to allow easy referencing at all times.

Conclusion

There are many ways that you can serve the disabled population in your fitness center. You need to decide how best to accommodate these needs, train your staff accordingly, and perhaps equip your site with a few pieces of wheelchair-accessible strength training equipment. For cardiovascular exercise, an arm ergometer can also be included.

Remember that no one is immune to the possibility of facing a disability at some point in time. A significant number of individuals every day find their lives suddenly impacted forever by spinal cord injury or illness. While the quality of these lives may be considerably altered, exercise can be a very positive and productive means of sustaining healthy and active lifestyles in the midst of a disabling condition. Whether the individual is motivated to strength train for better sports performance, the improved ability to conduct routine daily activities, assistance with weight management, maintaining muscle mass and bone density, or for various psycho-social reasons, the benefits are strongly associated with numerous aspects of health and wellness (Schulz and Decker 1985).

Through the use of innovative and accessible fitness equipment, safe and effective training techniques, educational resources, a knowledgeable staff, and a network of supportive health care professionals in your area, you can be well on your way to serving this most appreciative population.

The rewards of becoming involved in fitness training for the disabled will extend to everyone in your fitness center, including staff, members, volunteer trainers, program participants, and many in your community as well. You will find that as you serve in this capacity, *workouts on wheels* will inspire those involved to new levels of personal achievement and fulfillment.

The Training Protocol

Individuals in our program follow a two- or three-day per week exercise routine for about one hour per session. We adhere to the American College of Sports Medicine guidelines for strength training, which advocate slow, controlled movements (ACSM 1998). As mentioned earlier, slow movements are also helpful when working with individuals who exhibit higher levels of spasticity.

One set of eight to 12 repetitions is performed with a light weightload initially, to establish the proper settings at a conservative pace. If a participant cannot complete an exercise in good form in the 10- to 12-repetition range, the resistance should be reduced to accommodate the ability of the individual. While we advocate one-set training, if a participant is using exceptionally light weightloads we may opt to perform an additional set or two. Time constraints, however, are often a factor in this decision. Attaching wrist cuffs, positioning and securing the wheelchair properly, adjusting the exercise apparatus for each muscle group, and recording the training progress on a workout card take additional time and therefore make one-set training a practical choice.

A number of upper body exercises can be performed on the VersaTrainer. This apparatus is a strength training device for individuals in wheelchairs that uses power rods of various weights attached to a cable pulley system for resistance. The system facilitates bilateral or unilateral movements, and offers handgrips or wrist cuffs depending on the gripping ability of the exerciser. It is compact, easily adjustable, and requires no wheelchair transfers. The equipment comes with a detailed notebook and photographs explaining the exercises and demonstrating how to safely secure the wheelchair. Our training protocol typically includes the bench press, seated row, triceps extension, biceps curl, triceps dips, and shoulder shrugs. However, there are a number of additional exercises available. Depending on the ability and training interests of the participant, you can develop a program that is most suitable for his or her requirements. You may wish to train larger muscle groups first as you would for other exercisers, or for maximum efficiency, you may perform the exercises in an order that facilitates the frame adjustment of the equipment and the positioning of the wheelchair.

Wheelchair Stabilization

It is important that the wheelchair be secured before each exercise is performed. After establishing the proper position for your client, make sure the wheel casters are facing the footplates and lock the wheel locks. If the wheel locks are inadequate, or if the participant is using an athletic wheelchair without wheel locks, you may place sand weights at the front of the wheelchair and behind the wheels for greater security (Lockette et al. 1994). Additional stabilization may be accomplished by attaching the straps provided by VersaTrainer to the wheelchair and hooking them to the side rails, tightening them for a firm hold. A lap belt is also available. Grasp the hook of each side of the lap belt and attach to the left and right side bars respectively. Fasten the belt together and tighten snugly without restricting circulation. Redness of the skin, swelling, or a pins-and-needles sensation indicate that the belt should be loosened. It is also helpful to loosen straps between training sets (Lockette et al 1994).

The following exercises are grouped according to wheelchair positioning and are performed in this order by our participants.

Bench Press

The best exercise for developing overall upper body pushing strength, and addresses the pectoralis major, triceps, and anterior deltoids. Assists in wheelchair propulsion and transfers, and uses the pushing motion found in sports such as basketball.

Pulley Position:	Shoulder level.
Body Placement:	Participant's back to power rods, upper shoulders resting on support foam.
Starting Position:	Keep arms horizontal to the floor, elbows bent and held at shoulder level, forearms parallel to one another. Grasp the

handles, palms facing down.

Execution: Push handles away from chest, extending arms directly in front of the chest. The closer together the handles are, the more work is performed by the triceps muscles.

Breathing Technique: Breathe out on the pushing movement and breathe in on the return movement.

Triceps Extension

Strengthens the triceps muscles and stabilizes the elbow joint, which helps prevent injury. Beneficial for transfers, wheelchair propulsion and reaching overhead.

Pulley Position: Shoulder level.

Body Placement: Participant's back to power rods. Lock-down system secured.

Starting Position: Hold the upper arm horizontal, forearm vertical, and palm facing in at about ear level. The participant or trainer should stabilize the elbow of the arm to be exercised.

Execution: Extend forearm to a position parallel with the floor. Slowly return the forearm back toward the ear.

Breathing Technique: Exhale on the push; inhale on the return.

Resisted Dips

Works the pectoralis major, triceps and anterior deltoid muscles. Excellent for wheelchair sports such as road racing, basketball, or tennis. Also helpful for wheelchair transfers.

Pulley Position: Highest level.

Body Placement: Participant's back to power rods. Lock-down system secured.

Starting Position: Grasp handles. Upper arms should be almost parallel to the floor.

Execution: With palms facing in press downward toward the axle of the wheel or directly toward the floor. Slowly return to starting position.

Breathing Technique: Breathe out on the pushing movement and breathe in on the return movement.

Seated Row

Strengthens and stretches the latissimus dorsi, biceps, posterior deltoids, and rhomboid muscles. May also enhance natural breathing capacity and range of movement in the arms. Strengthens opposing muscle groups of wheelchair locomotion.

Pulley Position: Shoulder level.

Body Placement: Participant facing power rods, wheelchair positioned toward the back of the platform. Lock-down system

	secured.
Starting Position:	Reach forward and grasp both handles, palms facing down. Bring the torso upright to stabilize against the back of the wheelchair throughout the movement.
	Please Note: The participant may need assistance grasping the handles and returning to the upright position. To help maintain a stabilized trunk position, the trainer may place gentle pressure on the shoulders to hold firmly in place.
Execution:	With palms facing downward draw the arms toward the lower chest, turning the palms in toward the body halfway through the movement phase and maintaining this position as the palms are pulled close to the chest. Do not go beyond a perpendicular, erect upper body position when pulling the handles toward the upper chest. Slowly return to the starting position, bending slightly at the waist and *only* at the waist. This allows for greater range of motion and greater isolation of the latissimus dorsi.

Biceps Curl

Develops the biceps and forearm flexor muscles. Beneficial for daily life activities, wheelchair transfers and lifting objects.

Pulley Position:	Lowest level. Pulleys inverted.
Body Placement:	Participant facing power rods. Lock-down system secured.
Starting Position:	Stabilize arm performing the exercise by holding elbow with the opposite hand, or having the trainer hold elbow securely. Grasp handle, palm facing up, arm extended. The trunk should be upright and stationary.
Execution:	Pull handle up, curling the forearm toward the upper arm. Maintain a stable back and arm position; keep elbow stationary. Lower forearm slowly to starting position.
Breathing Technique:	Breathe out when pulling up toward the upper arm and breathe in when returning to starting position.

Shoulder Shrugs

Strengthens the upper trapezius and neck extensor muscles. Also helps increase shoulder stability, enhances posture and helps prevent injury.

Pulley Position:	Lowest level.
Body Placement:	Participant facing power rods. Lock-down system secured. Wheelchair positioned toward the back of the platform.
Starting Position:	Grasp handles, palms facing in toward the body. Sitting erect, the cables should be under tension.
Execution:	Roll shoulders forward, upward, and back slowly.

Maintain an erect position and keep shoulders under control. *Please note:* Participants may be tempted to use the elbows rather than the upper trapezius and neck extensor muscles to pull the cable upward. To prevent this, make sure the elbows do not bend in this exercise.

Breathing Technique: Breathe naturally, exhaling on the completion.

Sometimes a quadriplegic participant will prefer using accessible Nautilus machines that include the bench press, compound row, the biceps curl, and triceps press. If a participant has good upper body strength and is able to transfer onto the equipment with moderate assistance, secure the wheelchair as close to the equipment as possible, Lock-down system in place. As the participant positions his or her upper body and torso onto the equipment, gently move the lower body into place.

Nautilus Bench Press

This is the best exercise for developing overall upper body pushing strength, and works the pectoralis major, triceps, and anterior deltoids. Assists in wheelchair propulsion and transfers, and uses the pushing motion found in sports such as basketball.

Beginning Position: Lie with chest directly below handles. Grasp handles so that hands are positioned slightly wider than shoulder-width apart.

Execution: Press handles upward until elbows are almost fully extended. Return slowly to starting position and repeat. Remember to keep head and hips on the bench. Keep feet on floor or footrest.
Note: It may be necessary to gently stabilize the participant's feet and torso during this exercise, particularly if the lower body enters into some spastic movements.

Breathing Technique: Breathe out when pushing handles away from chest, and breathe in when returning to starting position.

Nautilus Compound Row

Strengthens and stretches the latissimus dorsi, biceps, posterior deltoids and rhomboids. May also enhance natural breathing capacity and range of movement in the arms. Strengthens opposing muscle groups of wheelchair locomotion.

Beginning Position: Adjust seat so handles are at shoulder level. Sit with chest against chest pad and torso erect. Place feet flat on floor. Grasp each handle, arms fully extended.

Execution: Slowly pull handles back toward chest. Keep wrists straight. Allow handles to return slowly until arms are fully extended.

Breathing Technique: Breathe out when pulling toward the chest and breathe in when returning to starting position.

Nautilus Biceps Curl

Strengthens the biceps and forearm flexor muscles. Beneficial for daily life activities, wheelchair transfers and lifting objects.

Beginning Position:	Adjust seat so elbows are in line with machine's axis of rotation, typically indicated by red dots, and upper arms are parallel to floor. Grasp handles with underhand grip, elbows slightly flexed. Sit with chest against chest pad, torso erect.
Execution:	Slowly curl handles upward until elbows are fully flexed. Keep wrists straight. Allow handles to return slowly to starting position.
Breathing Technique:	Breathe out when pulling handles up to full elbow flexion, and breathe in when returning to starting position.

Nautilus Triceps Press

Strengthens the triceps, pectoralis major and anterior deltoid muscles. Beneficial for transfers, wheelchair propulsion and reaching overhead.

Beginning Position	By squeezing the seat adjustment lever, position the seat so that shoulders are slightly above elbows while grasping the ends of the exercise handles. Secure the seat belt.
Execution:	Press the handles downward until elbows are almost fully extended. Return slowly to the starting position and repeat.
Breathing Technique:	Breathe out when pushing handles downward to full elbow extension and breathe in when returning to starting position.

Chapter 10

New Discoveries and Directions

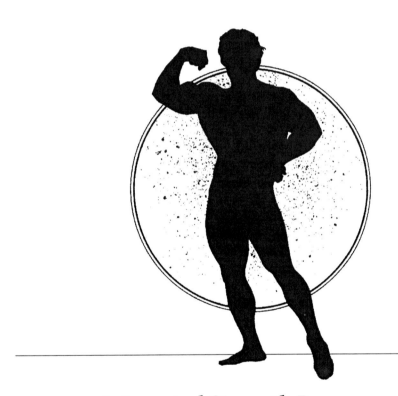

**Integrated Strength Programs
for Comprehensive Conditioning**

During the last few years, we have completed several studies on exercise factors related to strength development. These include the effects of combining strength training and endurance exercise, the effects of combining strength training and stretching exercise, training perceptions during the first several weeks of strength exercise, and strength training frequency. Based on the research results, we have developed recommendations for program design and implementation that should be useful for fitness professionals.

Strength Training and Endurance Exercise

During the past decade it has been widely accepted that strength training is the best means for improving muscular fitness and that endurance exercise is the best means for improving cardiovascular fitness (ACSM 1990). Most fitness facilities provide both strength equipment (e.g., Nautilus machines) and endurance equipment (e.g., treadmills, cycles, steppers, etc.), and most fitness professionals recommend both strength exercise and endurance exercise for their clients. Assuming that most fitness participants perform a combination of strength and endurance exercise during their training sessions, does the activity order have an effect on strength development?

To answer this question, we recently conducted four separate studies in which half of the subjects always performed strength training followed by endurance training, and half of the subjects always performed endurance training followed by strength training (Westcott and La Rosa Loud 1999). In each 10-week study, the strength training program consisted of 12 Nautilus exercises, performed for one set of eight to 12 repetitions each, and the endurance training program required about 25 minutes of continuous treadmill walking or stationary cycling at approximately 70 percent of predicted maximum heart rate.

Strength gains were assessed for different muscle groups in each of the four studies: study one examined changes in the 10-repetition maximum leg extension test (quadriceps); study two examined changes in the 10-repetition maximum chest press test (pectoralis major and triceps); study three examined changes in the 10-repetition maximum super pullover test (latissimus dorsi); and study four examined changes in the 10-repetition maximum lateral raise test (deltoids).

As you will note in Table 10-1, the strength gains were similar for both training protocols (strength exercise followed by endurance exercise and endurance exercise followed by strength exercise). In fact, the combined data for the 205 adult subjects who participated in these studies revealed essentially no difference in strength development due to activity order. As shown in Table 10-1, the subjects who always did strength exercise first experienced a 16-pound overall strength increase, and the subjects who always performed endurance exercise first experienced a 15-pound overall strength increase.

The findings from these studies revealed no difference in strength development due to activity order. In other words, whether participants perform strength

Study	A	B	C	D	ALL
Subjects	23	43	71	68	**205**
Muscles	Quadriceps	Pectoralis Major	Latissimus Dorsi	Deltoids	**Combined**
Strength First Group	+23 lbs.	+15 lbs.	+14 lbs.	+18 lbs.	**+16 lbs.**
Endurance First Group	+20 lbs.	+9 lbs.	+15 lbs.	+18 lbs.	**+15 lbs.**

Table 10-1   Changes in muscle strength for subjects who performed strength training followed by endurance exercise and subjects who did endurance exercise followed by strength training (205 subjects).

exercise followed by endurance exercise or endurance exercise followed by strength exercise appears to be a matter of personal preference.

It should be noted that the endurance training in these studies was performed at a moderate effort level (approximately 70 percent of predicted maximum heart rate), and for a moderate duration (about 25 minutes). It is possible that harder or longer endurance workouts may adversely affect a subsequent strength workout. Consequently, participants who perform more demanding endurance exercise may experience better muscular development by doing their strength training first.

Strength Training and Stretching Exercise

To determine the effects of combined strength training and stretching exercise we conducted three studies in which each Nautilus exercise was followed by a brief stretch for the target muscle group (Westcott and La Rosa Loud 2000a).

Study One: Strength and Stretching Exercise

In the first study, 15 previously untrained adults performed one set of 12 Nautilus exercises, eight to 12 repetitions each, two or three days a week for 10 weeks. A similar group of 19 adults followed the same strength training protocol, but performed a 20-second stretching exercise for the muscles just worked immediately after each Nautilus exercise. Both groups also did about 25 minutes of moderate effort aerobic activity (treadmill walking or stationary cycling at approximately 70 percent of predicted maximum heart rate) during each training session. As shown in Table 10-2, the subjects who did strength training without stretching exercise increased their muscle strength by 16.6 pounds (10-repetition maximum leg curl test), whereas the subjects who did strength training with stretching exercise increased their muscle strength by 20.5 pounds.

	Strength Only	Strength Training Plus Stretching
Study One (N = 34)	+16.6 lbs.	+20.5 lbs.
Study Two (N = 42)	+16.3 lbs.	+18.6 lbs.
Combined Results (N = 76)	+16.4 lbs.	+19.5 lbs.

Table 10-2   Changes in muscle strength for subjects who performed only strength training and subjects who did strength training plus stretching exercise (76 subjects).

Study Two: Strength and Stretching Exercise

In the second study, 21 previously untrained adults performed one set of 12 Nautilus exercises, eight to 12 repetitions each, two or three days a week for 10 weeks. A similar group of 21 adults followed an identical strength training program, but performed a 20-second stretching exercise for the muscles just worked immediately after each Nautilus exercise. Both groups also did about 25 minutes of moderate effort aerobic activity (treadmill walking or stationary cycling at approximately 70 percent of predicted maximum heart rate) during each training session. As presented in Table 10.2, the participants who did strength training without stretching exercise increased their muscle strength by 16.3 pounds (10-repetition maximum leg curl test), whereas the participants who did strength training with stretching exercise increased their muscle strength by 18.6 pounds.

The combined data for these two studies revealed a 16.4-pound strength gain for the 36 subjects who performed strength training without stretching exercise, and a 19.5-pound strength gain for the 40 subjects who did strength training with stretching exercise (see Table 10-2). Although the 19 percent greater strength gain did not reach statistical significance, it indicated a trend favoring strength training with stretching over strength training without stretching for strength development in beginning exercisers. In addition, the group that performed both strength training and stretching exercise increased their joint flexibility (sit and reach test) by 2.4 inches, compared to a 1.5-inch improvement for the group that did only strength training.

Study Three: Strength and Stretching Exercise

In the third study, 32 previously sedentary subjects performed 12 Nautilus exercises followed by a 20-second static stretch at the machine for the muscles just worked (distributed stretching). A similar group of 47 previously sedentary subjects performed the same strength training program, but did a consolidated sequence of six 20-second static stretches on a StretchMate apparatus during

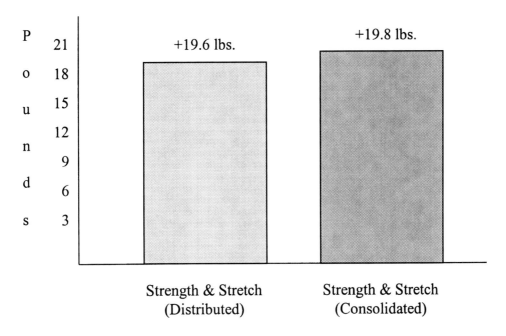

Figure 10-1   Changes in hamstring strength for subjects who did strength training plus distributed stretching and subjects who did strength training plus consolidated stretching (79 subjects).

each workout. As illustrated in Figure 10.1, the exercisers who did strength training and distributed stretching gained 19.6 lbs. in hamstring strength, and the exercisers who did strength training and consolidated stretching gained 19.8 lbs. in hamstring strength. This study showed no significant difference in strength gains for subjects who did distributed or consolidated stretching exercises.

The combined data for all three studies revealed a 16.4-pound strength gain for the 36 subjects who performed strength training without stretching exercise, and a 19.6-pound strength gain for the 119 exercisers who performed strength training plus stretching exercise (see Figure 10-2). These results further support the benefits of combined strength and stretching exercise. It is possible that stretching in conjunction with resistance training may make muscles more responsive to strength-building stimuli.

Based on these findings, we recommend a combined program of strength training and stretching exercises for enhancing both muscle strength and joint flexibility. Our preferred protocol is to follow each Nautilus exercise with a 20-second stretch for the muscles just worked. This strength-stretch pairing procedure has produced excellent results without increasing the overall workout duration. Because our members average about one minute of rest between Nautilus exercises, the 20-second stretches fit neatly into the non-training intervals. Appendix A illustrates the 12 stretching exercises our members perform in conjunction with their 12 standard Nautilus exercises.

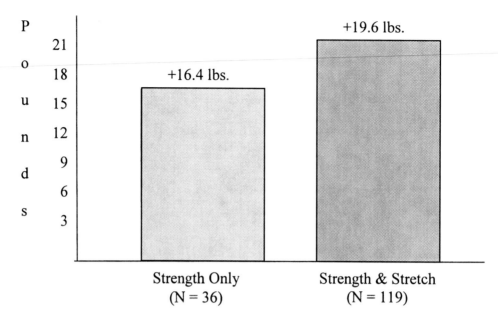

Figure 10-2   Combined results of hamstring strength gains for subjects who did strength training only and for subjects who did strength training plus stretching (155 subjects).

Perceived Exertion and Exercise Introduction

To learn more about beginners' response to strength training, we conducted a research project that examined the participants' perceived exercise exertion as they progressed through their first nine weeks of strength workouts. This study included 83 previously sedentary adults (average age 49 years) who performed a standard circuit of strength exercises two or three days a week. Each workout consisted of one set of eight to 12 repetitions on the following Nautilus machines: (1) leg extension; (2) leg curl; (3) chest cross; (4) decline press; (5) super pullover; (6) lateral raise; (7) biceps curl; (8) triceps extension; (9) low back; (10) abdominal; (11) neck flexion; and (12) neck extension.

As shown in Table 10-3 the subjects' average exercise weightloads (10 repetition maximum) increased from 43.4 lbs. (Week 3) to 51.6 lbs. (Week 6) to 55.6 lbs. (Week 9). On the same assessment days, their average perceived exertion ratings (Borg Scale) increased from 11.5 (Week 3) to 13.5 (Week 6) to 13.8 (Week 9). The Borg Scale begins at 6 (essentially no exertion) and ends at 20 (maximum physical effort).

These data revealed an almost parallel increase in strength development and training effort. This leads to the question of whether greater muscle strength results in greater exercise effort or whether greater exercise effort results in greater muscle strength?

Week	Mean Exercise Weightload	Mean Perceived Exertion	Borg Scale Rating
3	43.4 lbs.	11.5	Fairly Light
6	51.6 lbs.	13.5	Somewhat Hard
9	55.6 lbs.	13.8	Somewhat Hard/Hard

Table 10-3   Average exercise weightloads (10 repetition maximum) and perceived exertion ratings (Borg Scale) during the third, sixth, and ninth week of strength training (83 subjects).

On average, the new exercisers added 3.0 lbs. of muscle over the 9-week training period. Therefore, at least part of their strength gain could be attributed to more muscle. However, part of the strength gain could also be due to higher exercise effort as the participants progressed through the training program. That is, both physiological and psychological factors may influence strength development in beginning adult exercisers. Logically, it makes sense for new participants to start with relatively light weightloads and low effort, then progress gradually to higher levels of resistance and exercise exertion.

Week	3	6	9
Leg Extension	13.3	14.1	14.5
Leg Curl	12.1	12.9	13.3
Chest Cross	12.9	14.3	14.3
Decline Press	13.7	14.1	14.5
Super Pullover	12.3	13.5	14.1
Lateral Raise	12.5	13.4	13.8
Biceps Curl	13.0	14.1	14.7
Triceps Extension	13.0	14.1	14.4
Low Back	11.3	12.3	12.6
Abdominal Curl	12.4	13.6	13.4
Neck Flexion	11.3	12.8	13.2
Neck Extension	11.3	12.4	12.8

Table 10-4   Perceived exertion ratings on Borg Scale for 12 Nautilus exercises during the third, sixth, and ninth weeks of training (83 subjects).

In a second aspect of this study, the subjects rated the 12 machine exercises for performance effort as they completed one set of 12 repetitions to momentary muscular fatigue. As you can see in Table 10-4, their perceived exertion levels were consistently lower on the midsection and neck exercises and consistently higher on the leg extension and arm exercises, with the torso exercises generally rated between these effort levels.

Based on our reports, perhaps the first exercises we should introduce to new strength training participants are the low back and abdominal machines, followed by neck extension and neck flexion on the four-way neck machine. Without question, these are the most important muscles in the human body, as they control our posture, provide core strength, and protect against degeneration and injury to our spinal column. Clearly, this is a good place to start the strengthening process, and these exercises seem to be best accommodated by previously inactive adults.

After these machines are mastered, it makes sense to add the torso machines (chest cross, super pullover, lateral raise), as they were rated a little more physically challenging. Of course, other torso machines could be substituted if these exercises are not available.

The data indicates that it may be best to introduce the leg and arm exercises last, because the leg extension, biceps curl and triceps extension ranked highest in perceived exertion. Although the leg curl was considered easier to perform, we suggest teaching it with the leg extension in the final group of exercises.

To summarize, the previously sedentary adults' perceived exertion ratings indicate that this sequence of exercise introduction may enhance their strength training competence, confidence, and compliance:

Week 1:   Low back, abdominal, neck extension, neck flexion

Week 2:   Chest cross, super pullover, lateral raise

Week 3:   Leg extension, leg curl, biceps curl, triceps extension

Strength Training Frequency

Several years of studies with youth, adults, and seniors have shown that two strength training sessions per week are sufficient for attaining significant increases in muscle strength and mass (Westcott and Guy 1996). This is good news for many time-pressured people who have difficulty maintaining a three-day-per-week exercise program. Certainly, two 20-minute strength workouts a week represent a very time efficient training program. However, we have found that a considerable number of individuals who work long hours and/or two jobs are unable to set aside exercise time on weekdays. We therefore conducted a research study to compare the strength gains for subjects training one, two, or three days per week.

The participants in this program were 218 previously sedentary adults and seniors who enrolled in a 10-week beginning exercise program (mean age 50 years). During each activity session, the subjects performed about 25 minutes of strength training (12 standard Nautilus machines) and about 25 minutes of endurance exercise (treadmill walking or stationary cycling). One-hundred and three participants trained on Mondays, Wednesdays and Fridays, 86 participants trained on Tuesdays and Thursdays, and 29 participants trained only on Saturdays.

With respect to strength development, the three-day-per-week exercisers had a mean increase of 21.2 pounds, the two-day-per-week exercisers had a mean increase of 15.5 pounds, and the one-day-per-week exercisers had a mean increase of 15.5 pounds. All three training frequencies produced significant strength gains. Although they performed only two-thirds as much weekly exercise, the two-day trainees achieved 73 percent as much strength improvement as the three-day trainees. Remarkably, the one-day trainees also attained 73 percent as much strength development as the three-day trainees even though they performed only one-third as much weekly exercise.

While three strength training sessions a week may be most productive for beginning participants, the findings from this study suggest that one or two relatively brief bouts of strength exercise may be sufficient for stimulating significant strength gains in previously sedentary adults and seniors. These results are consistent with those in our study of young figure skaters reported in Chapter Five. Apparently, just one workout a week will produce impressive improvements in muscle strength when the exercises are performed with proper technique and to the point of temporary muscle fatigue.

Summary

Based on the studies presented in this section, it would appear that fitness participants may successfully combine strength training and endurance exercise as well as strength training and stretching exercise. We have found no differences in strength development between subjects who did strength training before endurance exercise and subjects who did endurance exercise before strength training. We therefore recommend that the activity order be a matter of personal preference.

Our research has indicated two benefits from integrating strength training and stretching exercise. Participants who performed a 20-second static stretch after each Nautilus exercise or who did six consolidated stretches on a StretchMate apparatus increased both joint flexibility and muscle strength more than subjects who did not stretch during their workout. We suggest that each Nautilus exercise be followed by a brief stretch for the muscle group just worked. This procedure addresses all of the major muscle groups, adds little, if any, time to the overall training session, and enhances both strength and flexibility development.

We found that previously inactive adults increased their muscle strength and their exercise effort during the first several weeks of strength training. Apparently, both physiological and psychological factors influence strength development in beginning exercisers. The same subjects reported lower levels of perceived exertion on the midsection and neck exercises, moderate levels of perceived exertion on the torso exercises, and higher levels of perceived exertion on the leg extension and arm exercises.

Practical Application

Although there are many ways to introduce strength exercises to new participants, the findings from these studies suggest that beginners may benefit from a program such as the following.

Week 1:

- Participants perform one set of 8 to 12 repetitions in the low back, abdominal, neck extension and neck flexion exercises.
- Participants do a 20-second static stretch for the muscles just worked following each strength exercise.
- Participants complete 10 to 15 minutes of treadmill walking, stationary cycling or other aerobic activity before or after the strength exercises.

Week 2:

- Participants perform one set of 8 to 12 repetitions in the chest cross, super pullover, lateral raise, low back, abdominal, neck extension and neck flexion exercises.
- Participants do a 20-second static stretch for the muscles just worked following each strength exercise.
- Participants complete 15 to 20 minutes of treadmill walking, stationary cycling or other aerobic activity before or after the strength exercises.

Week 3:

- Participants perform one set of 8 to 12 repetitions in the leg extension, leg curl, chest cross, super pullover, lateral raise, biceps curl, triceps extension, low back, abdominal, neck extension and neck flexion exercises.
- Participants do a 20-second static stretch for the muscles just worked following each strength exercise.
- Participants complete 20 to 25 minutes of treadmill walking, stationary cycling, or other aerobic activity before or after the strength exercises.

Weeks Following:

- After the third week of workouts, the training effort may be gradually increased for both the strength and endurance exercises.
- Generally speaking, the strength exercises should use sufficient resistance to fatigue the target muscles within 8 to 12 controlled repetitions. Whenever 12 repetitions can be completed in good form, the weightload should be increased by one to three pounds.
- As a rule, the endurance exercise should start with easy effort (warm-up phase), progress to moderate effort (approximately 65 to 75 percent of maximum heart rate), and finish with easy effort (cool-down phase).

Conclusion

This basic and brief program of integrated strength, flexibility and endurance exercise is the basis for the new *Nautilus Expressway Training Program.* Our research studies show major improvements in muscle strength, joint flexibility, cardiovascular endurance, and body composition (more muscle and less fat) when the training program incorporates these exercise components. Finally, just two or three days a week is all it takes to attain excellent results from this highly effective and efficient exercise program, and even one good strength workout per week may be sufficient for attaining significant physical benefits.

Exercise Descriptions and Illustrations

This section provides exercise descriptions and illustrations for the new 2ST line of Nautilus machines, as well as the at-machine stretching exercises. The instructions for proper use of each machine are concisely presented, and the desired movement patterns (beginning and ending positions) are clearly illustrated. Keep in mind that the most important consideration when performing rotary exercises, such as lateral raises, is to align the body axis of rotation with the machine axis of rotation. When doing linear exercises, such as overhead presses, set the seat for a full but comfortable range of joint movement. We recommend completing each repetition in a controlled manner, taking at least two seconds to lift the weightstack and four seconds to lower the weightstack.

Nautilus Exercise Machine Instructions

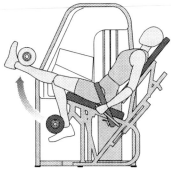

LEG EXTENSION

1. Sit on seat and place both legs behind adjustable movement pad.
2. Align both knees with machine axis of rotation (red dot), squeeze seat adjust lever to position seat back against your hips, and grip handles lightly.
3. Lift movement pad upwards until knees are straight, and pause momentarily.
4. Return slowly to starting position, and repeat.

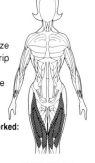

Major Muscles Worked:
Quadriceps

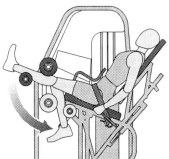

SEATED LEG CURL

1. Sit on seat, push the leg entry handle forward, slide your legs between the adjustable movement pads, and return the handle to its resting position.
2. Align both knees with the machine axis of rotation (red dot), squeeze the seat adjust lever to position the seat back against your hips, and grip the handles lightly.
3. Curl both legs to pull the movement pad towards your hips, and pause monetarily.
4. Return slowly to starting position, and repeat.

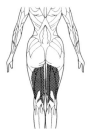

Major Muscles Worked:
Hamstrings

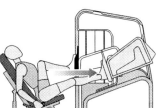

LEG PRESS

1. Sit with both feet evenly placed on footpad, heels at bottom.
2. Adjust seat so that thighs are close to chest and directly behind feet.
3. Push footpad forward until both knees are almost fully extended, but not locked out.
4. Return slowly to starting position and repeat.

Major Muscles Worked:
Quadriceps, hamstrings, gluteals

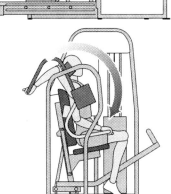

SUPER PULLOVER

1. Squeeze the seat adjust lever to sit with your shoulders in line with the machine axis of rotation (red dot).
2. Secure the seat belt and press the foot lever to position the movement pads.
3. Place your arms on the movement pads, grip the crossbar lightly with fingers, release the foot lever, and stretch your arms upward as far as comfortable.
4. Pull your arms downward until the crossbar touches your midsection, and pause monituarly, leaning forward slightly so low back touches seat back.
5. Return slowly to starting position, and repeat.
6. Press the foot lever, take your arms off the movement pads, release the foot lever gently, and exit the machine.

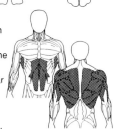

Major Muscles Worked:
Latissimus dorsi, teres major, rhomboids, middle trapezios, rectus abdominis, triceps, and rear deltoids

Nautilus Exercise Machine Instructions

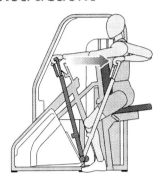

COMPOUND ROW

1. Squeeze chest pad adjust lever so hands just reach the handle when seated.
2. Squeeze seat adjust lever so arms are parallel to floor when seated.
3. Select preferred grip (vertical or horizontal) and pull handles backward to chest, and pause monituarly.
4. Return slowly to starting position and repeat.

Major Muscles Worked:
Latissimus dorsi, teres major, biceps, middle trapezius, rhomboids, rear deltoids

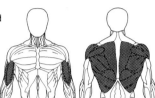

10° CHEST

1. Lie on back with head on bench and shoulders in line with red dots.
2. Place arms under roller pads, with hands open, facing away from weight stack.
3. Move roller pads up, touch together, and pause momentarily.
4. Return slowly to starting position

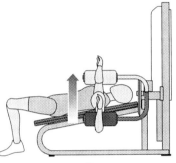

Major Muscles Worked:
Pectoralis major, anterior deltoids

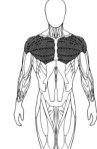

VERTICAL CHEST

1. Sit with shoulders approximately even with handles.
2. Place feet on footpad and press forward to position handles.
3. Grasp handles and release footpad.
4. Press handles forward until elbows are almost fully extended.
5. Return slowly to starting position and repeat.
6. After final repetition, place feet on footpad and press forward to reposition handles.

Major Muscles Worked:
Pectoralis major, anterior deltoids, triceps

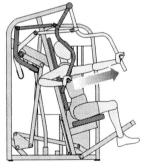

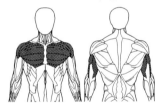

Major Muscles Worked:
Deltoids and upper trapezius

LATERAL RAISE

1. Squeeze the seat adjust lever to sit with shoulders in line with the machine axes of rotation (red dots).
2. Place arms against your sides inside the movement pads, and grip the handles lightly.
3. Lift the movement pads just above horizontal, and pause monetarily.
4. Return slowly to starting position and repeat.

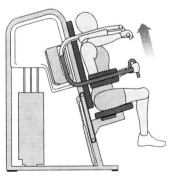

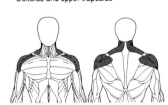

Nautilus Exercise Machine Instructions

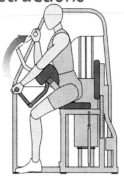

PREACHER CURL

1. Squeeze the seat adjust lever to sit with both elbows in line with the machine axis of rotation (red dot).
2. Partially stand, grip the movement bar loosely, and sit in the properly aligned position.
3. Curl the movement bar upward as far as possible, and pause monetarily.
4. Return slowly to starting position, and repeat.
5. Partially stand and lower the movement bar to its resting position to exit.

Major Muscles Worked:
Biceps brachli, brachialis, and forearm flexors

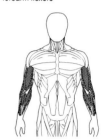

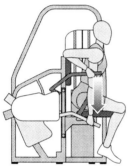

TRICEPS PRESS

1. Squeeze seat adjustment lever to sit with elbows slightly above shoulders while grasping handles.
2. Secure seat belt.
3. Press handles downward until elbows are almost fully extended.
4. Return slowly to starting position and repeat.

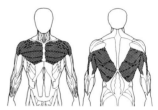

Major Muscles Worked:
Triceps, pectoralis major, pectoralis minor, latissimus dorsi, anterior deltoids

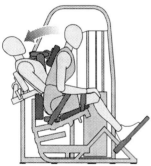

LOWER BACK

1. Squeeze the seat adjust lever to sit with your navel in line with the red dot, and your hips firmly against the seat back.
2. Position the foot pad so that your knees are a little higher than your hips, and secure the seat belts across your thighs and hips.
3. Push the movement pad backwards by contracting your low back muscles, and pause monetarily.
4. Return slowly to starting position, and repeat.

Major Muscles Worked:
Erector spinae

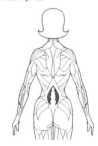

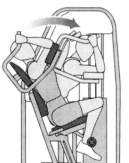

ABDOMINAL

1. Squeeze the seat adjust lever to sit with your navel in line with the red dot, and hook feet behind roller pads.
2. Place your elbows on the movement pads and grip the handles lightly with fingers.
3. Pull your chest towards your hips by contracting your abdominal muscles in a crunch movement, and pause monetarily.
4. Return slowly to starting position, and repeat.

Major Muscles Worked:
Rectus abdominis

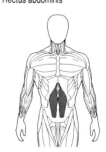

Nautilus At-MachineStretching Exercises

Leg Extension

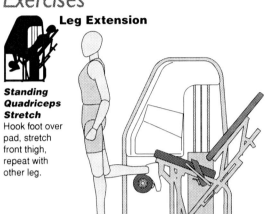

Standing Quadriceps Stretch
Hook foot over pad, stretch front thigh, repeat with other leg.

Super Pullover

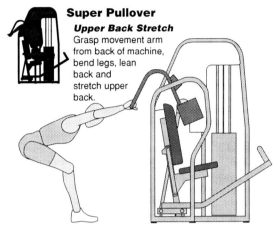

Upper Back Stretch
Grasp movement arm from back of machine, bend legs, lean back and stretch upper back.

Seated Leg Curl

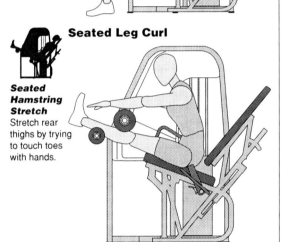

Seated Hamstring Stretch
Stretch rear thighs by trying to touch toes with hands.

Compound Row

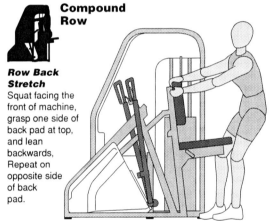

Row Back Stretch
Squat facing the front of machine, grasp one side of back pad at top, and lean backwards, Repeat on opposite side of back pad.

Leg Press

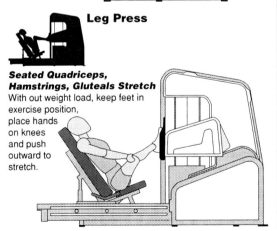

Seated Quadriceps, Hamstrings, Gluteals Stretch
With out weight load, keep feet in exercise position, place hands on knees and push outward to stretch.

10° Chest

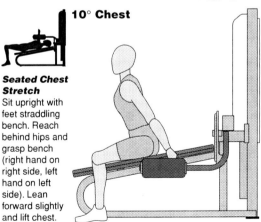

Seated Chest Stretch
Sit upright with feet straddling bench. Reach behind hips and grasp bench (right hand on right side, left hand on left side). Lean forward slightly and lift chest.

Nautilus At-Machine Stretching Exercises

Vertical Chest

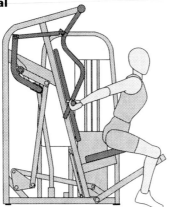

Vertical Chest Stretch
Sit upright on edge of seat. Reach back and grasp outside handles (right hand on right side, left hand on left side). Lean forward slightly and lift chest.

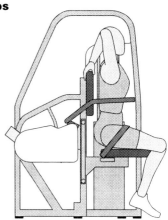

Triceps Press

Seated Triceps Stretch
After completing triceps press, lower seat all the way. Reach right hand over right shoulder and grasp top of back support pad. Stretch right triceps for 20 seconds, and repeat reaching left hand over left shoulder to grasp top of back support pad.

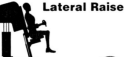

Lateral Raise

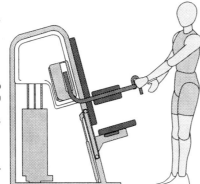

Standing Deltoid Stretch
Stand facing machine, grasp left handle with left hand and turn shoulders to the left. Repeat with right handle and right hand.

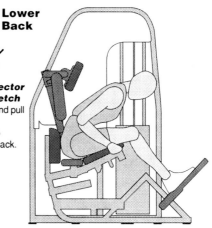

Lower Back

Seated Erector Spinal Stretch
Grasp seat and pull forward and downward to stretch low back.

Preacher Curl

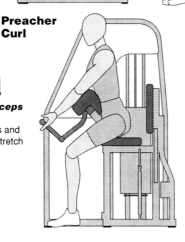

Seated Biceps Stretch
Extend arms and hands and stretch biceps.

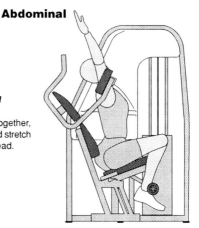

Abdominal

Seated Abdominal Stretch
With hands together, arch back and stretch arms over head.

Nutrition Topics and Handout Materials

This section presents the nutrition handouts provided each week to participants in the Workout For Weight Management Program. Special thanks to Rita La Rosa Loud, Program Director, and the following members of her staff for developing and compiling these materials: Katrina Armstrong, Edyce Binder, Heather Chandor, Kathy Clark, Karen Leary, Chris McDonough, Kathy Pavlopoulos, Sheryl Rosa, Donna Serino, and Skip Tull.

The Food Guide Pyramid

The Food Guide Pyramid provides healthful and helpful guidelines for daily food choices. The base of the Pyramid includes breads, cereals, rice, and pasta. The next level includes both fruits and vegetables. You need servings of all these foods in your diet to provide carbohydrates, vitamins, minerals, and fiber. The milk, yogurt, and cheese group along with the meat, poultry, fish, dry beans, eggs, and nuts group make up the third level. Foods from these groups are important for protein, calcium, iron, and zinc. The fats, oils and sweets that make up the tip of the Pyramid provide lots of calories and little to no nutrients.

The number of servings you need from each group depends on how many calories you use daily. You should have at least the lowest number of servings in each range. The following suggestions are for only three calorie levels. If you fall between levels, estimate servings between the suggested numbers.

	About 1,600 Calories	About 2,200 Calories	About 2,800 Calories
Bread Group Servings	6	9	11
Vegetable Group Servings	3	4	5
Fruit Group Servings	2	3	4
Milk Group Servings	2-3	2-3	2-3
Meat Group (ounces)	5	6	7
	About right for many sedentary women and some older adults.	About right for most children, teenage girls, active women, and many sedentary men.	About right for teenage boys, many active men, and some very active women.

Table B-1   The Food Guide Pyramid

So now that you know how many servings you should have, you need to know what counts as a serving.

Bread, Cereal, Rice and Pasta Group

1 slice of bread	1/2 of bagel
1/2 cup of cooked pasta	3-4 small crackers
1/2 cup of cooked rice	1 oz. breakfast cereal

Vegetable Group

1/2 cup cooked
1 cup leafy, raw
1/2 cup non-leafy, chopped, raw

Fruit Group

1 whole fruit
1/2 cup canned
3/4 cup fruit juice

Milk, Yogurt and Cheese Group

1 cup skim milk, whole milk	1/2 cup ice cream or frozen yogurt
8 oz. Yogurt, lowfat, nonfat	2 oz. processed cheese

Meat, Poultry, Fish, Dry Beans, Eggs, and Nuts Group

1 egg - 1 oz.	2 T. peanut butter - 1 oz.
lean meat, poultry, fish,	1/2 cup dry beans - 1 oz.
cooked - 3 oz.	

Table B-2   What Counts as a Serving?

Fats *"use sparingly"*	Watch out for hidden fats (e.g., salad dressings, toppings, baked goods, and processed foods). However, remember fats should be included in a balanced diet. A good rule of thumb for those who overindulge is to reduce the amount of fat intake. If you are one of those who has close to or completely cut out fats, increase fat intake.
Dairy Group *2-4 servings*	Choose dairy products that are low in fat and sodium. You'll be surprised how many choices there are. For example, a low fat alternative to ice cream is non fat yogurt or sorbet.
Meat Group *2-3 servings*	Choose leaner meats and be sure to remove skin and trim any visible fat before cooking. Tuna packed in water is a better option than packed in oil. Remember, white meat has less fat than dark meat. All natural brands of peanut butter have less sugar and contain the healthier fats. Beans and legumes are also an excellent source of protein.
Vegetable Group *3-5 servings*	Choose a variety of vegetables to balance nutrients. Dark leafy green vegetables are richer in nutrients than iceberg. Steam, microwave or stir fry veggies to minimize loss of vitamins and minerals and try eating raw veggies more often. Especially when you're hungry, reach for veggies as a snack.
Fruit Group *2-4 servings*	Like vegetables, a variety of fresh fruits are a great source of fuel for the body. They make great snacks too. Although fruit juices can be counted as a serving of fruit, beware of the high sugar content. Fresh fruit from the vine are preferable. Dried fruits are also a good source of fiber and nutrients but can add up to a significant amount of calories (for example, 12 raisins is equivalent to 1 medium apple).
Grain Group *6-11 servings*	Breads and grains make up the base of the Food Pyramid Guide. Whole grain breads, brown rice, and pastas are higher in fiber than enriched white flour products. Eating foods high in fiber plays an important role in stabilizing the blood sugar and prevents cravings.
Water	Drink water regularly throughout the day. Eight cups of water is the minimum amount of fluid recommended. Drink before and after meals, especially before, during and after exercise to replace fluids lost. Water adds to satiety and energizes the body. Try adding a twist of lemon or lime for added flavor.

Table B-3   Food Pyramid Guide Serving Recommendations

Workout for Weight Management Menu Plan

For those who are diet oriented or considered "professional dieters", the Workout for Weight Management Menu Plan is not a diet in the traditional sense of the word. Think of this plan as a life style change whether you need to lose weight or not.

The Workout for Weight Management 8 week menu plan and calorie breakdown is based on the Food Guide Pyramid serving recommendations. The number of servings you need daily depends on your activity level. Choose the menu plan that best suits your lifestyle.

Calorie Breakdown

1,600 calories

About right for many sedentary women and some older adults

2,200 calories

About right for most children, teenage girls, active women, and many sedentary men

2,800 Calories

About right for teenage boys, many active men, and some very active woman

Menu Planner

The menu planner helps you keep track of the number of servings. Check off each food item as you consume them. Each week you will be provided a sample meal plan for a typical day and a recipe of the week. The recipes of the week are designed to please your whole family so you don't have to cook two meals in order to follow the meal plan. The recipes of the week include chicken, fish, turkey, pork, pasta beef and vegetarian meals.

Design your own meal plan by using the serving numbers as a guide. For example, you may exchange servings from meal to meal (save your meat servings all for dinner instead of splitting the servings lunch and dinner). When preparing food avoid deep frying. Try to broil, roast, oven fry, bake or grill. Also, trim all visible fat and remove skin on meat.

How you can have more spreads and toppings

By using the lower fat versions of foods it allows you more freedom with your meal plan (using a fat free cream cheese on your bagel will not use up one of your fats from your plan allowing you to use a fat during another meal). On the next page are some examples. Just go to your local supermarket and compare nutrition labels.

	Calories	Fat
mayonnaise, regular 1 T	100	11
mayonnaise, lite 1 T	44	4
mayonnaise, fat free 1 T	10	0
cream cheese, regular 1 oz	99	10
cream cheese, lite 1 oz	62	5
salad dressing, regular 1 T	69	7
salad dressing, lite 1 T	16	1.5
salad dressing, fat free 1 T	30	0
cream cheese, fat free 1 oz	25	0

Table B-4   Spreads and Toppings

Beverages

Excluding milk, water, diet drinks, coffee and tea. For purposes of weight loss, it is highly recommended to avoid high calorie beverages such as regular soda, sweetened juice, alcohol, etc., which should be counted as one serving in the Fats, Sweets, and Oils category.

Combined Foods

To incorporate combined foods such as pizza, pasta dishes, frappes, and casseroles, all it takes is a little thought. If you prepare the meal just pay close attention to the measurements of major ingredients such as milk, meat, fats and veggies. When ordering do like the rest of us and request ingredients amounts from the wait staff.

Calories and Portion Control

The trend toward lowfat eating can be seen in just about every supermarket and convenience store today with nonfat yogurt and milk all the way to lowfat cookies. However, we have become so focused on fat content that we may have forgotten one other very important component, calories.

Calories tell us how much energy we get from food. Whether that food is a banana or a piece of cake, our bodies either use those calories right away or store them, mainly as fat. The bigger the portions we eat, the more calories we take in, the more fat we store. It really is as simple as that.

Portion sizes in restaurants have grown huge. It's not unusual for an appetizer and dinner to total over 2,000 calories, which for many people would be their total calorie intake for the whole day! Sandwiches bought from a deli can contain as much as 8 ounces of meat, more than twice a recommended serving size, and some fat-free muffins and bagels are so huge they contain up to 700 calories! This trend towards large portions may be rubbing off on meals served in the home too. After drinking those super huge soft drinks we get at the movies, a regular juice glass at home begins to look tiny!

This does not mean, however, that we can all just forget about fat. One gram of fat contains more than twice the amount of calories as a gram of protein or carbohydrate which means that a lowfat diet can help you cut back on calories. But as well as fat, you need to look at calories and portion sizes to help control your weight.

Helpful Tips for Portion Control

To help you start taking control of your daily portions, here are some helpful tips:

Eating at Home

- One cup of cereal should fill half a typical cereal bowl.
- One portion of mashed potatoes should be the size of your fist.
- A serving of meat should be about the size of a deck of cards.
- Serve meals on smaller plates. This helps you adjust to smaller servings but your plate is still "full."

Dining Out

- If you know you're going out for dinner, eat a light lunch.
- Don't count on a restaurant portion as a serving. Figure you're getting at least twice the amount that is considered a serving on the USDA Food Guide Pyramid.
- Order items that are poached, steamed, or baked. They tend to be low in fat and have fewer calories.
- Split an entree with your dining partner or request half an order for yourself.
- If you're served a large portion, immediately ask for a takeout box and put half of your meal in it to enjoy tomorrow!

Carbohydrates—The Base of the Pyramid

Consuming 60% of your daily calories from carbohydrates is what most experts recommend. Why is that? Good question. Since carbohydrates are the main source of fuel for your body (brain and muscle cells) they should be the basis of your diet. The more active you are the more carbohydrates you need. Let's see how it all fits together.

Simple and Complex Carbohydrates

There are two types of carbohydrates, simple and complex. Simple carbohydrates or sugars include glucose, fructose, and galactose. These three sugars combine to produce other common carbohydrates, such as maltose (starch in grains), sucrose (table sugar), and lactose (sugar in dairy products).

Chemically speaking, complex carbohydrates are formed when simple sugars bind together in a long chain. Your body then converts both complex carbohydrates (starch) and simple sugars that you've eaten to glucose and uses these sugars to produce energy.

Because the body stores relatively little glucose in the liver and in the muscles it is essential to consume adequate amounts of carbohydrates in your diet every day to replenish the energy you expend. Your activity level determines the amount of carbohydrates you need to function optimally on a daily basis. Sound complex? It's really very simple.

Which of the Carbohydrates is most useful?

Most experts suggest the complex kind for getting through the day's activities and providing the body with nutrients it needs to perform at its best. One concern with eating mostly carbohydrates is whether you will gain weight. Carbohydrates are not fattening; but an excessive intake of any food category can lead to a weight gain. Consider what you put on the top of your breads, pasta and potatoes, and you may notice that it's not the carbohydrates but the high-fat toppings like oil, cream cheese and gravy that add up in calories.

Another problem with carbohydrates is that your blood sugar will rise rapidly on a diet that is comprised mostly of simple sugars, especially if you eat them all at once. Your pancreas will secrete insulin, a hormone whose main function is to lower or normalize your blood sugar level. The fact that your body is capable of using only small amounts of glucose at a time forces some of the glucose to be stored as fat. When the brain senses a rapid rise in blood sugar it may release too much insulin, which lowers blood sugar and may cause cravings for more sugar. Increased consumption of complex carbohydrates can help prevent this problem. Nutrient rich complex carbohydrates are easily digested in the intestines and enter the bloodstream more slowly than simple sugars. Good sources of complex carbohydrates include grains, vegetables, legumes (beans and peas) and fruits, all found at the base of the Food Pyramid Guide, as well as lowfat dairy products.

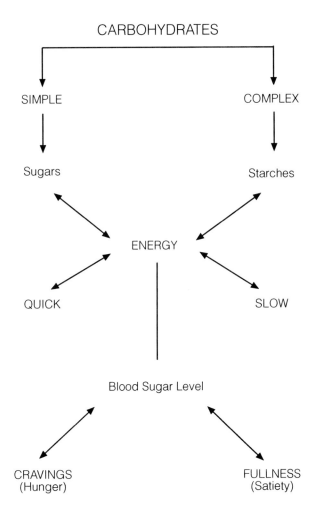

Figure B-1   Carbohydrates

Protein: How Much Do You Need?

It should be noted that excessive amounts of protein do not enhance muscle strength. There is no scientific data stating that protein intakes exceeding 0.9 grams/lb. of body weight will provide an additional advantage to athletes.

Why do you need protein?

You need protein to build and repair your muscle tissue, grow hair and fingernails, produce hormones, boost your immune system and replace your red blood cells.

	Grams of Protein per Pound of Body Weight
Current RDA for sedentary adult	0.4
Recreational exerciser, adult	0.5 - 0.75
Competitive athlete	0.6 - 0.9
Growing teenage athlete	0.8 - 0.9
Adult building muscle mass	0.7 - 0.9
Athlete restricting calories	0.8 - 0.9
Maximum usable amount for adults	0.9

Table B-5   How much protein do you need?

Problems associated with too much protein

- People who eat too much protein may eat too little carbohydrate to fuel their exercise energy requirements.
- Excess protein leads to an increased need to urinate, which increases the risk of becoming dehydrated and becomes burdensome to the kidneys.
- A diet high in protein tends to be high in fat.

Protein Supplements

Protein powders and amino acid pills have been promoted as essential for optimal muscle development. It should be kept in mind that larger muscles result from strength training rather than food supplements.

	Grams of Protein/Standard Serving
Animal Sources	
egg white	3.5 per 1 large egg
egg	6 per 1 large
cheddar cheese	7 per 1 oz.
milk, 1%	8 per 8 oz.
yogurt	11 per 1 cup
cottage cheese	15 per 1/2 cup
haddock	27 per 4 oz. cooked
hamburger	30 per 4 oz. broiled
pork loin	30 per 4 oz. roasted
chicken breast	35 per 4 oz. roasted
tuna	40 per 6 oz.
Plant Sources	
almonds, dried	3 per 12 nuts
peanut butter	4.5 per 1 tablespoon
kidney beans	6 per 1/2 cup
hummus	6 per 1/2 cup
refried beans	7 per 1/2 cup
lentil soup, Progresso	11 per 10.5 oz.
tofu, extra firm	11 per 3.5 oz.
baked beans	14 per 1 cup

*Data from Nancy Clark's Sports Nutrition Guidebook, 2nd Edition, 1997. Human Kinetics.

Table B-6   Sources of Protein

Fear of Fat: The Good, The Bad, The Deceiving

Which end of the Fat Spectrum do you dominate? Do you tend to over-indulge in your fat intake by eating lots of sweets and drinking whole milk dairy products? Or are your shelves filled with fat-free and lowfat foods in order to keep your daily intake of fat to less than 10%? It seems that Americans just aren't comfortable consuming 20-30% of their calories from fat and tend to dominate each end of the fat spectrum.

% Daily Intake of Fat

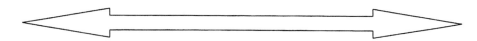

0%   5%   10% 15% 20% 25% 30% 35% 40% 45% 50% 55% 60%

Where do you belong on the Fat Spectrum?

You know that fats contain twice as many calories per gram as carbohydrates or protein (fats = 9 grams, carbohydrates = 4 grams, and protein = 4 grams). But wait! This doesn't mean that you should cut fats completely out of your diet. Fats have some major responsibilities to carry out within the body. Fats provide the body with energy, provide insulation against temperature extremes, supply protection against shock, insulate the nerves, transport fat-soluble vitamins (A,D,E, and K), slow digestion and add satiety and a sense of fullness. Therefore, some fats are essential such as monounsaturated and polyunsaturated fats, while others such as saturated fats and trans fat should be strictly limited in your diet. Total fat intake should be less than 30 percent of your daily calories.

Classification of Fats

The Good:
Unsaturated Fatty Acids

1. Monounsaturated fatty acid (MUFA):

   Monounsaturated fats should be one of the major sources of fat in your diet. However, most experts say that MUFA should not exceed 15 percent of our daily calories. Foods that contain MUFA are olives, olive oil, canola oil, peanut oil, almonds, macadamia nuts and natural peanut butter. Replacing saturated fatty acids with MUFA will help reduce low density lipoprotein cholesterol (*bad* cholesterol) as well as total cholesterol.

2. Polyunsaturated fatty acid (PUFA):

   Increased amounts of PUFA also actively lower serum cholesterol and low density lipoprotein cholesterol concentration (*bad* cholesterol).

PUFA is another major source of fat in your diet which should not exceed 10 percent of your daily calories. PUFA is found in oils that are liquid at room temperature such as corn, sunflower, soybean, sesame and safflower oil. Mayonnaise and soft margarine are other sources. The essential PUFAs found in these foods are omega 6 and omega 3 fatty acids. Deficiencies of PUFA may produce growth retardation, reproductive failure, skin abnormalities, and kidney and liver disorders.

The Bad:
Saturated Fatty Acids

Saturated fats found in animal foods tend to raise blood cholesterol, one of the major risk factors for heart and artery disease. Coconut and palm oil are a source of saturated fat even though they are of vegetable origin. Generally, the more saturated a fat, the firmer it is. For example, butter is harder than margarine because butter is saturated and margarine, unsaturated. Other sources of saturated fat include whole milk dairy products, egg yolks, and chocolate. You want to restrict these fats to less than 10 percent of your total daily calories.

The Deceiving:
Trans Fat

Trans fat is found in margarine, deep-fried foods and prepared foods such as baked goods and snacks. Foods that are "cholesterol free," "low cholesterol," "low-saturated fat" or made with vegetable oil aren't necessarily low in trans fat. But saturated-fat-free foods are. Are you confused? That is why trans fat is so deceiving. Trans fat, like saturated fats, raises your bad cholesterol. But trans fat also lowers your *good* cholesterol, unlike saturated fatty acids. Remember, the less fat in a food means less trans fat.

How to Avoid Trans Fat

- Look for foods that contain no vegetable shortening or partially hydrogenated oil.
- Avoid deep-fried foods.
- Choose lower-fat margarines, chips, crackers, cookies, and pastries (if you must eat them).
- Use olive oil and canola oil instead of butter, margarine, or shortening.
- If you use margarine, buy tubs rather than sticks. Get light, lowfat, or fat-free brands.

Removing Fat From Foods Cuts Calories

1. Eliminate fat as a seasoning and in cooking.
2. Choose meats carefully. Select lean cuts.
3. Eat meat infrequently and in small amounts.

4. Replace high-fat foods with lowfat alternatives.
5. Emphasize fruits and vegetables.

Reducing Fat Consumption Will Result In

1. Lower LDL-C (*bad* cholesterol) and total cholesterol levels.
2. Lower caloric intake.
3. Lower fat weight.

The Sat Fat Switch

Switch from	Switch to
Meat, Poultry, Seafood	
Hamburger, meatloaf	Ground turkey breast, veggie burger
T-bone, rib eye, prime rib	Round steak, sirloin
Pork chops, ribs	Pork Tenderloin
Regular hot dog, bologna, sausage	Fat-free or lowfat hot dog, bologna, sausage
Poultry with skin	Skinless poultry
Fried chicken or fish	Broiled, grilled or roasted chicken or fish
Chicken thigh, wing	Chicken breast, drumstick
Dairy Products	
Whole or 2% fat milk	1% or skim milk
Regular cheese	Reduced-fat or lowfat cheese
Regular ice cream	Lowfat or fat-free ice cream or frozen yogurt
Regular cream cheese	Light or fat-free cream cheese
Sweets and Desserts	
Cheesecake, cheese danish, croissant, brownie, pie, donut, poundcake...	Fruit, dried fruit or small serving of lowfat sweet (sherbert or sorbet...)
Snacks	
Chocolate bar, sandwich crackers, bugles, popcorn popped in coconut oil	Fruits, vegetables, whole-grain crackers, "light" popcorn, pretzels, baked potato chips, rice cakes
Condiments	
Butter or margarine, sour cream	Whipped light butter, lower-fat tub margarine, fat-free or lowfat sour cream

Water: The Most Important Nutrient

Although water has no calories or nutrients, it is essential for all life processes to occur. An average adults' body weight is comprised of 60% water. Generally, the proportion is relative to lean body mass therefore, an athlete's percentage of water will be higher than that of an obese person. Every aspect of body function is impaired by not drinking enough water. The body constantly attempts to restore homeostasis by adjusting water balance (intake/outtake) and its distribution. Water is vital for proper absorption, digestion, excretion, circulation and joint lubrication. It also acts as a solvent for minerals, vitamins, amino acids, glucose, etc., and as a regulator of body temperature and blood volume.

How much water is really necessary?

The basic recommendation is eight 8 ounce cups of water daily, because we typically lose that much through vapor from the lungs, sweat from the body, and excretion. This must be replenished for appropriate water balance. Although our minimum water requirement is approximately 8 cups, physical activity and warm weather increase our fluid needs. An increase in protein or salt in our diets also requires more water to maintain electrolyte balance, and to help the kidneys flush out excess salt and waste products of protein metabolism.

Are there other ways to satisfy proper fluid requirement other than plain or fancy waters?

Yes. Other fluids are fine and can be consumed by drinking milk, fruit juices, lemonade, soup, etc. Consider the moisture content of these representative foods.

Lettuce, cucumber, tomato	95%
Orange	85%
Banana	75%
Beef, Chicken	60%
Cheese	35%
Cookie	5%

Sports drinks also provide fluids along with carbohydrates and electrolytes. They are typically high in calories, but may be an excellent choice during long and strenuous workouts.

What about caffeinated drinks?

Because coffee, tea and soft drinks act as a natural diuretic they are less desirable rehydration sources. The same is true for alcoholic drinks. It is recommended that for every caffeinated drink, you should consume the same amount of water.

Is thirst a good indicator for fluid replenishment?

Not necessarily. Your body requires fluids prior to the point of thirst. The sensation of thirst is caused by an abnormally high concentration of sodium in the blood resulting from dehydration. The thirst mechanism becomes less reliable as we age, so older adults should drink water frequently even though they do not feel thirsty.

What happens to the body when we don't supply it with enough water?

Water balance is critical to maintaining blood volume which affects blood pressure.

Dehydration

- decreases blood volume
- decreases oxygen to blood
- decreases urine output
- decreases blood pressure
- decreases nutrients to muscles
- decreases sweat
- increases heart rate
- increases body temperature
- tendency for muscle cramps
- kidneys retain water and sodium
- possibility of heat stroke
- possibility of heat exhaustion

Water Tips and Facts

- Fluids should be accessible at all times. Make this a habit.
- Practice drinking during exercise.
- Prehydrate 2 hours pre-exercise.
- In hot weather drink cool fluids to cool off faster.
- For every caffeinated or alcoholic drink, consume 1 cup of water.
- Sports drinks also help to prevent dehydration and are specifically formulated for electrolyte replacement.
- One medium mouthful equals 1 ounce.
- Reduce sweat loss by dressing appropriately. Wear white and light weight clothing during the summer. Wear layers you can discard during the winter exercise sessions.
- Monitor urine color. Dark indicates dehydration with a high concentration of metabolic waste. Clear indicates normal water balance and homeostasis.
- Drink water if you feel sluggish or fatigued.
- Increase intake of water dense foods such as fruit and vegetables.

Facts on Fiber

Dietary fiber is an important nutritional component that may help fight major health concerns, such as gastrointestinal disorders, heart disease and colon cancer. However, according to the National Cancer Institute, the majority of Americans are consuming only about half, or 15 grams of the recommended 20-30 grams of fiber we need on a daily basis.

Fiber is found in the structures of plants, such as stems, roots and leaves. We find fiber-rich foods in the grains category as well as fruits and vegetables. They are natural sources of complex carbohydrates and help give food shape, structure and bulk.

The Bulk of the Matter

- Fiber can be divided into two main categories: soluble and insoluble. Soluble fiber is found in citrus fruits and apples as well as in oats, navy, pinto and lima beans, barley and legumes. All of these help in lowering blood cholesterol, delaying glucose from being absorbed too quickly and regulating the digestive process.

- Insoluble fiber is found in wheat (bran), whole-grain breads and cereals, strawberries and raspberries, the skins of fruits and vegetables and poppy and sesame seeds. This form of fiber or roughage accelerates gastrointestinal transit, adds substance and bulk and assists in waste elimination.

- Both forms of fiber are broken down in the large intestine (this may lead to a feeling of fullness, distress or distention in the abdominal area). They also hold water and regulate bowel activity.

- Because of the length of time required for breakdown, fiber can delay the absorption of other nutrients. Please note it is important to drink plenty of water during the day and with meals, to help in digestion and offset this effect.

Amazing Grains: The Healthy Side of Fiber

- Insoluble fiber may help fight cancer by decreasing the levels of some toxins in the body.

- Fiber aids in weight control, because foods high in fiber are usually low in fat.

- High fiber diets are associated with low blood cholesterol which helps lower the risk of heart disease.

- Green and yellow leafy vegetables as well as citrus fruits offer protection against some forms of cancer.

- Lower rates of diabetes have been found in populations with higher carbohydrate diets.

Increasing Dietary Fiber

1. Eat berries, strawberries and raspberries.
2. Eat beans and corn.
3. Choose dark green, leafy forms of lettuce.
4. Look for 100% whole wheat when choosing breads.
5. Add high fiber cereals to your breakfast routine.
6, Eat the skins of potatoes.
7. Use whole wheat flour and brown rice.
8. Add wheat bran, oat bran and wheat germ to baked goods, cereals and yogurts.
9. Snack on dried fruits, which are concentrated forms of nutrients and fiber.
10. Instead of drinking juices, eat oranges, apples and grapes. Juices can also be high in sugar.

University of California at Berkeley Wellness Letter, April 1997.

Understanding Food Labels

Beware—and be aware!

Recently at my favorite supermarket I noticed a woman shopping with her teenage daughter. Both were wearing lycra tights, warm-up jackets and running shoes, but neither looked in particularly good shape. Little did I know that the next few minutes would provide me with an advanced course in deceptive packaging, misleading and confusing labeling, and outright false advertising.

It was obvious that this mother was trying to do the right thing, but with all the labels reading "light" this and "low" that, "reduced," "fortified", "natural", "organic," or "lean" she would have been better served with a dictionary than a shopping list.

Nutrition labeling can be very confusing, so we may need to dig a little deeper to learn what is really in the package. First, ignore the "Big Health Claim" on the front of the package (lite, cholesterol-free, contains oat bran, etc.). Turn it over and look for the ingredients and nutritional information usually listed on the side or back.

Nutritional labels tell you serving size, number of calories, and how much protein, carbohydrates, cholesterol, sodium and fat are in a serving of the product. The percent of Daily Value is also included and will help you interpret how foods will fit into your daily diet. But keep in mind that these percents are based on a 2,000 calorie/day diet so your daily values may be higher or lower depending on your calorie requirements. In general, try to attain the following percentages.

• Fat:	15-20%
• Carbohydrates:	60-70%
• Protein:	15-20%

Also included on the label is sodium content. Recommended daily allowance of sodium is less than 2400 mg.

If the nutritional information is listed, FDA regulations require that seven key vitamins and minerals be included on the label in a specific order, with corresponding percentages of the recommended daily allowance. Listings of 12 other vitamins and minerals, cholesterol, fats, and fiber, are optional. Ingredients are listed in descending order according to weight.

Labeling Terminology and Definitions

Contains no cholesterol:
But could be loaded with cholesterol-producing saturated fats.

Cholesterol-free:
Less than 2 mg cholesterol per serving.

Low cholesterol:
20 mg cholesterol per serving than regular version.

Low in saturated fat:
1 gram of saturated fat or less per serving.

Cholesterol reduced:
75% less cholesterol per serving than regular version.

Lowfat:
3 grams of fat or less per serving.

Lean:
A serving of meat and poultry with less than 10 grams of fat, less than 4 grams of saturated fat, and less than 95 mg of cholesterol per serving.

Extra lean:
Meat and poultry with less than 5 grams of fat, less than 2 grams of saturated fat, and less than 95 mg of cholesterol per serving.

Lite/Light:

An altered product containing 1/3 fewer calories or half the fat of the standard food. Also may describe the color or texture of the food.

High Fiber:

No standard definition. Also note, bran muffins are often loaded with saturated fat.

Low calories:

40 calories or less per serving.

Reduced calories:

At least 25% less calories per serving than the regular version.

Dietetic or diet:

Low or reduced calorie unless otherwise stated; may refer to low sodium.

Fortified:

Vitamins, minerals and protein added to food that naturally contains these in low amounts or not at all.

Imitation:

Resembles but contains fewer vitamins/minerals or less protein than the "regular" product.

Natural:

Meat and poultry with no artificial colors, flavors or preservatives, and minimally processed. A natural flavor comes from a plant or animal (sugar is a natural product).

Organic:

Some states require no pesticides to be present in fertilizer used to grow crops, or in the feed and water given to livestock. Otherwise, term has no definition.

Low sodium:

140 mg of sodium or less per serving.

No salt added:

Processed without salt but may contain sodium from other sources, e.g. MSG or soy sauce.

Reduced Sodium:

At least 75% less salt per serving than the regular version.

Very low sodium:

35 mg or less of salt per serving.

Sodium/salt free:

Less than 5 mg per serving of salt.

Sugar free/sugarless:

Less than 0.5 grams of sugar per serving.

Facts About Fat Substitutes

There are three kinds of fat substitutes currently manufactured.

- Carbohydrate Based—These are used in lowfat sauces, dressings, frozen desserts, and baked goods. They provide 4 calories per gram compared to the 9 calories per gram fat provides. Unfortunately these types of substitutes are destroyed by heat, which limits their use.

- Protein Based—(Brand name Simplesse) This fat substitute is created by specially processed egg and milk proteins. Since it is made from milk proteins it may cause allergic reactions for those who are sensitive to milk or eggs. Simplesse is used in lowfat baked goods, creamers, ice cream, cheeses, sour cream, spreads, dressings, soups, and sauces. Like the carbohydrate based substitutes, it provides 4 calories per gram, but is destroyed by heat.

- Chemically Changed Fat—(Brand name Olean, better known as Olestra) Olestra is made from vegetable oil and sugar, which create a complex structure that cannot be broken down or absorbed by the body. This is what makes Olestra fat-free. It is used in potato chips, crackers, tortilla chips, and other snacks. Unlike other fat substitutes Olestra is heat stable and can be used as a cooking oil. Products made with Olestra have the same taste and texture of the full fat counterparts.

Fat Substitutes Concerns

What is confusing to consumers is that some lowfat products have as many calories or close to as many as the full fat version. Also, many people see lowfat or fat-free on a label and use that as an excuse to eat more of that food. The could explain why some studies show that when people who eat high-fat diets incorporate lowfat foods into their eating plan only a moderate weight loss results, about 2 to 7 pounds. Unless a calorie deficit is created, which means using more calories than you eat, weight loss will not be achieved.

Olestra has two unique concerns. It may decrease the body's absorption of vitamins A, D, E, and K, the fat soluble vitamins, eaten around the same time the Olestra is ingested. The companies that use Olestra in products fortify them with the four vitamins to offset the problem. Also, since Olestra cannot be broken down by the body, it passes through unchanged creating similar results as high fiber foods. This effect of Olestra varies among people.

Replacing high-fat foods in your diet with the fat-free versions can help reduce your total daily fat intake and may reduce your risk of high-fat diet related diseases. Still the best way to achieve a healthy diet is to eat a variety of foods from the Food Guide Pyramid.

Fat Replacers You Can Use at Home

- Replace oil with applesauce in baked goods
- Replace oil with prune puree (sold as Sweeter Bake) in baked goods
- Use egg beaters or egg whites instead of whole eggs in recipes
- Use tofu to replace cheese in lasagna, and even cheesecake!

References

Facts About Olestra, American Dietetic Association, Web site www.eatright.org.

Roberts S. Zavier Pi-Sunyer F, et al. Physiology of Fat Replacement and Fat Reduction: Effects of Dietary Fat and Fat Substitutes on Energy Regulation. Nutrition Reviews 1998;56:S29-S38.

Soy Products

If you've heard about soy recently but are not familiar with this food, here is some basic information about soy products.

What Is Soy?

Soy products come from the soybean, which is native to eastern Asia. Soybeans contain many of the vitamins and minerals we need, such as iron, folic acid, calcium, magnesium, potassium, and the B vitamins. Soy is great for vegetarians because it is a non-meat product and has many of the good qualities that meat does. For example, it has a high protein value.

What is Beneficial About Soybeans?

Soybeans are low in saturated fat (the bad fat) and in total fat. They are cholesterol-free and very high in fiber. Many soy products contain isoflavons, which may work in several ways to help prevent certain diseases. Also soybeans are the base of many foods like tofu, soy nuts, soymilk, soy flour, and tempeh, which can all be used in different ways to add variety and new flavor to your meals and snacks.

What Are the Different Types of Soy Products?

Soy products can be found in simple forms such as soynuts, or in complex forms such as meat analogs. Below are definitions of various soy products.

The Bean: Whole soybeans (fresh) look like green peas. Dried soybeans have light tan or yellow color to them.

Soynuts: Whole soybean, dry-roasted, which can be eaten as a snack.

Soymilk: Rich milk made with soybeans and water. It is available in regular lowfat, and nonfat. Also available in many flavors, including natural, vanilla, chocolate, or carob. Soymilk is fortified with calcium and vitamin D and can be substituted for regular milk.

Soy Flour: Finely ground, roasted soybeans. Available in full fat and lowfat. Soy flour contains no gluten, therefore can only be partially substituted (5-25%) for wheat flour in baking.

Tofu: Soybeans that are pressed and cooked. Tofu is available in silken, soft, and firm forms. By having different textures, you can incorporate tofu into many recipes. The silken form can be added into soups and creams, the soft form as stuffing for shells or substitute for cheese, and the firm form as replacement for meat products or for imitation egg salad. Tofu acts like a sponge, so even though in the original form it tastes bland, once the sauce, herbs, and spices are added, absorption occurs and the tofu takes on the taste you give it.

Tempeh: Chunky, tender, cake made with soybeans and rice. The mixture is fermented to create a chewy texture and mild, smoky flavor. Tempeh can be barbecued or added in a cheese and tomato sandwich.

Miso: Smooth, salty paste with a tangy flavor usually used in soups, sauces and salad dressings.

Meat Analogs: Textured soy protein, dehydrated soy flour, and other ingredients, made to mimic meat and meat products. Some examples are hot dogs, ground beef, sausage, bacon, and pepperoni. All meat analogs are lower in fat than meats, but are available in lowfat and nonfat varieties.

What is Soy Powder and Textured Soy Protein?

These are all protein isolates, which means that they contain the largest amount of protein of all soy products. Soy powder is a powder that can be added to hot cereal, pudding, yogurt, cottage cheese, shakes and casseroles, to increase the protein value of the food. Textured soy protein or TSP has a texture similar to ground beef. It is de-fatted soy flour and it is sold in dry form. All it needs is rehydration and can be used as a substitute for ground meats.

Where Can Soy Products Be Bought?

The following chart will help you find soy products, tell you the supermarket section where they are usually located, or where else you can go to purchase them.

Soy product	Where to buy
Tofu	Produce or dairy, vacuum packed
Tempeh	Produce or dairy, vacuum packed, rectangle patties or cakes
Meat Analogs	Produce, dairy, freezer
Soymilk	Baked goods, dairy or health foods, non-refrigerated in boxes or powder form, or refrigerated in milk containers
Soy Flour	Baked goods/flour aisle
Textured Soy Protein (TSP)	In grain bins at health food stores or freezer section
Soy Powder	Health food section of supermarket or in nutrition and vitamin section in health food stores

Will My Family Like Soy?

Unless you make the first step to try soy products you will never know if you or your family will like it or not. Most soy recipes do not taste any different than the normal recipe. It might be easier to fit soy into your breakfast and lunch, instead of the main family meal which is usually dinner.

Cookbooks for Great Soy Cooking

The following are names of great cookbooks that incorporate soy into anything from a regular meal to a dessert.

New Soy Cookbook: Tempting Recipes for Tofu Tempeh, Soybeans & Soymilk by Lorna Sass and photographed by Jornelle Weaver (Chronicle Books, 1998).

The Soy Gourmet: Improve Your Health the Natural Way With 75 Delicious Recipes by Robin Robertson (Plume Publishing, 1998).

Soy of Cooking: Easy-To-Make Vegetarian, Low-Fat, Fat-Free & Antioxidant-Rich Gourmet Recipes by Marie Oser (Chronimed Publishing, 1996).

Information taken from Shape Magazine, March 1999, article entitled, "Soy Barrier", page 132 and from "Take 5 for Soy" by Erin Coffield, R.D.

Healthy Shopping Tips

First take a good hard look at what's in your kitchen cabinet and refrigerator. Do the foods you stock measure up to the five food groups of the Food Guide Pyramid? What can you do to build a healthy pantry?

Being label savvy is the first step to good nutrition. Make sure the products you plan to purchase aren't mostly added sugars. It's right on the label. Next, check the total amount of fat grams listed as well as the saturated fats, (the "bad" fats).

Supermarket Smarts

Tips for helping you get on the road toward a healthful diet:

- Keep the Food Guide Pyramid foremost in your mind when preparing your shopping list.
- Eat a healthy snack before you go grocery shopping. Never shop for food when you're hungry.
- Gravitate toward the healthy food section. Healthy foods are usually stocked around the perimeters of most supermarkets.
- When shopping, begin with the base of the Food Pyramid Guide— breads, cereals and grains. These are the foundation of most meals and should constitute the largest percentage of calories consumed.

- Following are nutritional breakfast, lunch and dinner suggestions from each of the five food groups:

Breads and Grains (6 to 11 servings)

Breakfast

Oats, wheat, barley, hot cereals (like oatmeal and cream of wheat), mixed grains, cold cereal (made from whole grains), bagels

Lunch

Whole wheat and pita bread, lowfat granola bars and crackers, wheat germ, pasta, pretzels

Dinner

Pasta, whole grain rolls and breads, brown, white or wild rice, bread sticks

Fruits and Veggies (3 to 5 servings)

Breakfast

Banana, peach, berries, apples, oranges, tangerines, grapefruit, grapes, melons, strawberries, cherries

Lunch

Carrots and celery sticks, salads, fresh fruit, steamed veggies

Dinner

Spinach, tomatoes, broccoli, string beans, asparagus

Meat Group (2 to 3 servings)

Breakfast

Eggs, egg whites, egg beaters, natural peanut butter

Lunch

Lean meat (95% fat free deli meats), tuna in water, legumes (chick peas, kidney beans, hummus), veggie burgers, lean or dark meats (less than 5 grams of fat)

Dinner

Poultry (chicken or turkey), red or black beans, fresh fish (swordfish, haddock), tofu and tempeh

Milk Group (2 to 3 servings)

Breakfast, Lunch, Dinner

1% skim milk, soy or rice milk, yogurt (plain or fruit flavored), lowfat cheese, cottage cheese and lowfat milk

Fats (use sparingly)

At the tip of the Food Guide Pyramid there are some fats that are healthier than others. Examples are olive, safflower, canola, flaxseed, sesame, walnut and peanut oils.

Be Prepared

Now that we've provided you with some healthy food choices, we'll offer you some preparation tips:

1. Add fruits and nuts to your hot or cold cereals (increases fiber, vitamins and minerals).
2. Keep cut up veggies in your fridge. You can easily grab them when you're hungry, pack them for lunch, or throw them into a saute for dinner.
3. Make a hearty salad filled with fruits, veggies, and legumes.
4. Add wheat germ to your yogurt to boost your protein, fiber, and overall energy.
5. For lack of refrigeration, fresh fruit, lowfat granola bars, boxed juices (100% fruit), lowfat cookies (Fig Newtons) and roll-ups are nutritious options for filling in the gap between meals.

Healthy Snacking

Do you ever find yourself skipping breakfast or lunch, or eating on the run? While watching T.V. or just before bedtime, do you feel a "snack attack" coming on? If you answer "yes", chances are you are among the 40 percent of harried Americans who munch and crunch small amounts of food throughout the day.

Although many people think of snacks as something extra they should not be eating, snacking can offer many benefits. For one, healthy snacking can help you to control your weight. Try thinking of snacks as mini-meals instead of extra treats that keep you from feeling too hungry. Eating several well-balanced snacks a day serve as building blocks to a healthy diet and make it easier to keep from overeating. Let the Food Pyramid be your guide. Select the larger percentage of your snacks from the base of the Pyramid (grains, fruits, and vegetables) and limit your intake of fats, oils, and sweets.

Because of our hectic lifestyles and schedules, many of us lack the time to sit down and eat three "square" meals a day. Snacking can be an effective solution to this problem by providing essential calories and nutrients otherwise missed by skipping meals. The trick is to avoid snacks high in calories, fat, and salt.

Taste is the most cited reason why certain snacks are selected. The most popular snacks are salty and crunchy, and are usually eaten in the afternoon and evening.

Indulging in a snack now and then is one of life's pleasures. Nutritious snacking in moderation is a habit one develops to nourish and sustain the body. Making snacking a healthy part of your lifestyle requires choosing snacks that promote dietary management and not sources of excess calories and fat. The answer is to select a variety of snacks from each of the

5 food groups making snacking a part of a balanced diet. Consider the following snack suggestions from the American Dietetic Association.

Salty

Baked or lowfat chips	Popcorn	Pretzels
Bread sticks	Lowfat crackers	String cheese

Crunchy

Apple	Popcorn	Raw vegetables
Baked or lowfat chips	Pretzels	(carrots, celery,
Bread sticks	Lowfat crackers	cauliflower, broccoli)

Sweet

Angel food cake	Fig bars	Sandwich cookies
Animal crackers	Frozen juice bars or	Vanilla Wafers
Applesauce	popsicles	Sugar-free jam or
Frozen yogurt, low fat	Fruit (fresh, dried,	jelly on toast, English
	canned)	muffin, or bagel

Lower Fat and Lower Calorie Choices

Grains
- Select lower fat grain products more often than higher fat choices
- Choose whole grain products to boost your fiber intake
- Choose enriched or whole grain products for B vitamins and iron.
- Pack cereal, crackers and rice cakes in single-serve containers for easy snacking on the run.

Fruits and Vegetables
- Most fresh fruits are portable and can be stored at room temperature for short periods of time without spoilage.
- Dried fruits are light-weight and resistant to spoilage.
- Buy canned fruit in single-serve containers.
- Pack fresh cut vegetables in zipper-lock storage bags.

Guidelines for Selecting Snacks (continued)

Milk, Yogurt, Cheese

- Select lower fat milk products more often than higher fat choices.
- Buy single-serve cartons of yogurt, cottage cheese, and pudding.
- Look for individually-wrapped cheese sticks and slices.
- Milk products require cold storage to prevent spoilage and foodborne illnesses.

Milk, Poultry, Fish, Eggs, Dry Beans, and Nuts

- Select lower fat meat and poultry products and use higher fat choices sparingly.
- Processed meats (luncheon meats, hotdogs) tend to be high in sodium.
- Meat products require cold storage and special handling to prevent spoilage and dangerous foodborne illnesses.
- Make trail mix with peanuts, raisins, pretzels, and dry cereal.

Guidelines for Selecting Snacks *(The American Dietetic Association)*

Workout on Wheels Program Materials

This section provides sample medical history, program application and volunteer application forms that may be useful in your program for individuals with disabilities. The medical history form is specifically targeted to people with spinal cord injury, as this is the primary focus of the chapter, *Workout on Wheels*.

Partnership Program Application

Date: _____

Contact Person _____

Day Phone ( ) _____ Evening Phone ( ) _____

Participant Name _____ Date of Birth _____

Address _____ City _____ State ___ Zip _____

Day Phone ( ) _____ Evening Phone ( ) _____

Disability(ies) _____

_____

_____

_____

Restrictions/Limitations _____

_____

_____

_____

Physical Therapist (PT) _____

Phone ( ) _____ Ext ___ Address _____

City _____ State _____ Zip _____

Occupational Therapist (OT) _____

Phone ( ) _____ Ext ___ Address _____

City _____ State _____ Zip _____

Personal Care Attendant (PCA) _____

Phone ( ) _____ Ext ___ Address _____

City _____ State _____ Zip _____

Participant Hours/Days Available to Train _____

_____

Medical Clearance? _____Yes _____No _____Pending

P.T. Exercise Prescription? _____Yes _____No _____Pending

O.T. Exercise Prescription? _____Yes _____No _____Pending

Medical History Questionnaire? _____Yes _____No _____Pending

Interests:

_____Cardiovascular Exercise   _____Treadmill

_____Versatrainer   _____Saratoga Cycle Ergometer

_____Track _____Equalizer 1000

_____Stationary Upright Cycle _____Pool (Ext 107)

_____Upright Chair _____Recumbant Cycle

_____Nautilus _____Gymnasium

_____StairMaster _____Freeweights _____Other

Cardiovascular Equipment:

Saratoga Cycle _____

Treadmill _____

Upright Cycle _____

Recumbent Cycle _____

StairMaster _____

Nautilus Machines:
Please attach a copy of the participant's Nautilus workout card indicating which exercises are being performed. If wheelchair transfers are necessary, please initial here that both the participant and volunteer have been trained in proper transfer technique. _____

Free Weights:
Please attach a copy of the participant's free weight workout card indicating which exercises are being performed. If wheelchair transfers are necessary, please initial here that both the participant and volunteer have been trained in proper transfer technique. _____

I, _____ , agree to participatate in the South Shore YMCA Partnership Program according to the guidelines established by my physician, physical therapist, occupational therapist and master trainer

_____
Participant Signature   Date

I, _____ , feel that I have been properly trained on the above equipment and feel confident in carrying out _____ 's training program.

_____
Volunteer Instructor Signature   Date

The participant and volunteer instructor have been trained on the proper use of the above equipment to the best of my knowledge.

_____
Master Trainer Signature   Date

Partnership Program Medical History Questionnaire

Name _____ Age _____ Date _____

Address _____ Phone _____

To assist us in designing the best possible fitness program for you, please answer the following questions regarding medical contraindications.

1. Please explain the nature of your disability.
2. What is the level of injury to your spine?
3. Is your injury complete or incomplete?
   If incomplete, please explain your left- and right-side movement abilities and sensation levels.
4. Are you presently in any pain? Please explain.
7. Do you have difficulty breathing?
8. Do you have pressure sores?
9. Do you experience heat or cold sensitivity?
10. Do you have full range of motion in your joints?
11. Do you experience spasticity?
12. Have you ever experienced throbbing headache, forehead sweating, goosebumps and/or a stuffy nose accompanied by very high blood pressure?
13. Do you have any bowel or bladder concerns?
14. Do you have any history of heart disease?
    Please explain.
15. Do you have any history of high blood pressure?
    Are you currently taking blood pressure medication?
16. Have you been diagnosed with diabetes or epilepsy?
    Are you currently taking medication?
17. Are you presently being treated by a physician or taking any medication(s)?
    If so, please list all medications.
18. Please describe your present level of fitness (poor, fair, average, above average).
19. Do you participate in sports activities?
20. What are your fitness goals?

South Shore YMCA Volunteer Application Form

Date: _____
Name: _____ Social Security #: _____
Address: _____
City: _____ State: _____ Zip: _____
Home Telephone: _____ Work Telephone: _____

Are you a member of the South Shore YMCA?   Yes_____ No_____
What services are you interested in volunteering?
How did you learn about the volunteer program?
    Staff_____ Y Member_____ Brochure_____
When are you available for volunteer service? Please provide days and
    time.
Have you done volunteer work in the past?   Yes_____ No_____
    Indicate agencies, dates and type of work:

Why do you want to volunteer for the South Shore YMCA?

Are there medical or other limitations to the type of volunteer work you
    could perform? Please explain.

Do you have your own transportation?Yes_____ No_____
What are your interest, skills and/or hobbies:

Educational Background:
High school: Major/Degree received:
College: Major/Degree received:
Other: Major/Degree received:

Work and/or volunteer references (list in order starting with most recent)
Company name and address:
    Supervisor's name, title, phone:
    Paid or volunteer/Reason for leaving:
    Brief description of responsibilities:
Company name and address:
    Supervisor's name, title, phone:
    Paid or volunteer/Reason for leaving:
    Brief description of responsibilities:
Company name and address:
    Supervisor's name, title, phone:
    Paid or volunteer/Reason for leaving:
    Brief description of responsibilities:

Personal References
Name, address, phone:
Name, address, phone:
Name, address, phone:
May we contact the references listed above?

Applicant's signature: _____

Partnership Program Volunteer—Reference Check

Applicant name: Phone:

Reference name: Phone:

Date:

How do you know the applicant?

How long have you known the applicant?

How would you rate the applicant in the following areas:

    Reliability:

    Judgment/Common Sense:

    Communication Skills:

    Works well with others:

    Initiative:

Is there any reason they might not be appropriate for a volunteer position working with the disabled?

STANDARD NAUTILUS
AND FREE WEIGHT EXERCISES

Standard Nautilus Machine and Free-Weight Exercises for the Major Muscle Groups.

Muscle Groups	Nautilus Machines	Free Weight Exercises
Quadriceps	Leg Extension Leg Press	Squat Lunge Step Up
Hamstrings	Leg Curl Leg Press Hip Extension	Squat Lunge Step Up
Hip Adductors	Hip Adduction	Ankle Weight Adduction
Hip Abductors	Hip Abduction	Ankle Weight Abduction
Gastrocnemius/ Soleus	Calf	Heel Raise
Pectoralis Major	Chest Cross Chest Press Bench Press Incline Press Weight-Assisted Bar Dip	Bench Press Incline Press Bar Dip
Latissimus Dorsi	Super Pullover Compound Row Weight Assisted Chin-Up	Pullover Bent Row Chin-Up
Deltoids	Lateral Raise Overhead Press Incline Press	Lateral Raise Overhead Press Incline Press
Biceps	Biceps Curl Weight-Assisted Chin Up	Biceps Curl Chin Up
Triceps	Triceps Extension Triceps Press Weight-Assisted Bar Dip	Standing Extension Lying Extension Bar Dip
Lower Back	Low Back	Trunk Extension
Rectus Abdominis	Abdominal	Trunk Curl
Obliques	Rotary Torso	Trunk Curl with Twist
Neck Extensors	Neck Extension	Shrug
Neck Flexors	Neck Flexion	———

American Association of Cardiovascular and Pulmonary Rehabilitation (1995). *Guidelines for Cardiac Rehabilitation Programs,* 2nd edition. Champaign, IL: Human Kinetics

American College of Sports Medicine (1990). The recommended quantity and quality of exercise for developing and maintaining cardiorespiratory and muscular fitness in healthy adults. *Medicine and Science in Sports and Exercise,* 22: 265-274.

American College of Sports Medicine (1998). The recommended quantity and quality of exercise for developing and maintaining cardiorespiratory and muscular fitness, and flexibility in healthy adults. *Medicine and Science in Sports and Exercise,* 30 (6): 975-991.

Ballor, D. and Poehlman, E. (1994). Exercise training enhances fat-free mass preservation during diet-induced weight loss: a meta analytic finding. *International Journal of Obesity,* 18: 35-40.

Brehm, B. and Keller, B. (1990). Diet and exercise factors that influence weight and fat loss. *IDEA Today,* 8: 33-46.

Butler, R., W. Beierwaltes, Rogers F. (1987). The cardiovascular response to circuit weight training in patients with cardiac disease. *Journal of Cardiopulmonary Rehabilitation* 7: 402-409.

Cahill, B. (Editor) (1988). *Proceedings of the Conference on Strength Training and the Prepubescent.* Chicago, Illinois: American Orthopaedic Society for Sports Medicine.

Campbell, W., Crim, M., Young, V., and Evans, W. (1994). Increased energy requirements and changes in body composition with resistance training in older adults. *American Journal of Clinical Nutrition,* 60: 167-175.

Darden, E. (1987). *The Nautilus Diet.* Boston: Little, Brown and Company.

DeMichele, P., Pollock, M., Graves, J., et al. (1997). Isometric torso rotation strength: Effect of training frequency on its development. *Archives of Physical Medicine and Rehabilitation,* 78: 64-69.

Draovitch, P. and Westcott, W. (1999). *Complete Conditioning for Golf.* Champaign, Illinois: Human Kinetics.

Drought, J. (1995). Resistance exercise in cardiac rehabilitation. *Journal of Strength and Conditioning* 17 (2): 56-64.

Evans, W. and Rosenberg, I. (1992). *Biomarkers.* New York: Simon and Schuster.

Faigenbaum, A., et al. (1990). Physiologic and symptomatic responses of cardiac patients to resistance exercise. *Archives of Physical Medicine and Rehabilitation* 70: 395-398.

Faigenbaum, A., Westcott, W., La Rosa Loud, R., Long, C. (1999). The effects of different resistance training protocols on muscular strength and endurance development in children. *Pediatrics,* 104 (1): 1-7.

Faigenbaum, A., Westcott, W., Micheli, L., Outerbridge,, A., Long, C., LaRosa Loud, R., and Zaichkowsky, L. (1996). The effects of strength training and detraining on children. *Journal of Strength and Conditioning Research,* 10 (2): 109-114.

Faigenbaum, A., Zaichkowski, L., Westcott, W., Micheli, L., and Fehlandt, A. (1993). The effects of a twice-a-week strength training program on children. *Pediatric Exercise Science,* 5: 339-346.

Feigenbaum, M. and Pollock, M. (1999). Prescription of resistance training for health and disease. *Medicine and Science in Sports and Exercise,* 31 (1): 38-45.

Fiatarone, M., Marks, E., Ryan, N., et al. (1990). High-intensity strength training in nonagenarians. *Journal of the American Medical Association,* 263 (22): 3029-3034.

Forbes, G. B. (1976). The adult decline in lean body mass. *Human Biology,* 48: 161-173.

Frontera, W., and Meredith, C., O'Reilly, K. et al. (1988). Strength conditioning in older men: Skeletal muscle hypertrophy and improved function. *Journal of Applied Physiology,* 64 (3): 1038-1044.

Ghilarducci, L., Holly, R., and Amsterdam, E. (1989). Effects of high resistance training in coronary heart disease. *American Journal of Cardiology.* 64: 866-870.

Gross, M., Roberts, J., Foster, J., Schankardass, K., and Webber, C. (1987, March). Calcaneal bone density reduction in patients with restricted mobility. *Archives of Physical Medicine and Rehabilitation,* 68: 158-161.

Hargrove, T. (1996). Study: Nearly 75 percent in United States are overweight. *The Patriot Ledger* (November 26). Quincy, Massachusetts.

Harris, K. and Holly, R. (1987). Physiological response to circuit weight training in borderline hypertensive subjects. *Medicine and Science in Sports and Exercise,* 19: 246-252.

Hurley, B. (1994). Does strength training improve health status? *Strength and Conditioning Journal,* 16: 7-13.

Hurley, B., Hagberg, J., Goldberg, A., et al. (1988) Resistance training can reduce coronary risk factors without altering VO_2 max or percent body fat. *Medicine and Science in Sports and Exercise,* 20: 150-154.

Jones, A., Pollock, M., Graves, J., et al. (1988). *Safe, Specific Testing and Rehabilitative Exercise For Muscles of the Lumbar Spine.* Santa Barbara, California: Sequoia Communications.

Kaplan, P., Roden, W., Gilbert, E., Richards, L. and Goldschmidt, J. (1981). Reduction of hypercalcurria in tetraplegia after weight-bearing and strengthening exercises. *Paraplegia,* 19 (5), 289-293.

Kelemen, M., et al. (1986). Circuit weight training in cardiac patients. *Journal of the American College of Cardiology* 7:38-42.

Keyes, A., Taylor, H. L. and Grande, F. (1973). Basal metabolism and age of adult man. *Metabolism,* 22: 579-587.

Koffler, K., Menkes, A., Redmond, W. et al. (1992). Strength training accelerates gastrointestinal transit in middle-aged and older men. *Medicine and Science in Sports and Exercise,* 24: 415-419.

Lockette, K. and Hayes, A. (1994). *Conditioning With Physical Disabilities,* Human Kinetics, Champaign, IL. Excerpts from www.GetFit.com.

Martinez, C. (1999). Exercise programming. *Fitness Management,* 15 (13): 36-37.

McCarthy, J., Agre, J., Graf, B., Pozniak, M., Vailas, A. (1995). Compatability of adaptive responses with combining strength and endurance training. *Medicine and Science in Sports and Exercise,* 27 (3): 429-436.

Menkes, A., Mazel, S., Redmond, R. et al. (1993). Strength training increases regional bone mineral density and bone remodeling in middle-aged and older men. *Journal of Applied Physiology,* 74: 2478-2484.

Miller, P., Editor (1995). *Fitness Programming and Physical Disability,* Human Kinetics, Champaign, IL.

Morris, F., Naughton, G., Gibbs, J., et al. (1997). Prospective ten-month exercise intervention in premenarcheal girls: Positive effects on bone and lean mass. *Journal of Bone and Mineral Research,* 12 (9): 1453-1462.

National Spinal Cord Injury Association (1999). *Spinal Cord Injury Statistics,* Fact Sheet #2, website http://www.spinalcord.org/resource/Factsheets/factsheet2.html.

National Spinal Cord Injury Association (1999). *Common Questions About Spinal Cord Injury,* Fact Sheet #1, website http://www.spinalcord.org/resource/Factsheets/factshee1.html.

National Strength and Conditioning Association (1995). Position paper on prepubescent strength training. *National Strength and Conditioning Association Journal,* 7:27-31.

Nelson, M., Fiatarone, M., Morganti, C., et al. (1994). Effects of high-intensity strength training on multiple risk factors for osteoporotic fractures. *Journal of the American Medical Association,* 272 (24): 1909-1914.

New York Times News Service (1991). "Considering a diet plan? Forget it, say experts," April 2.

President's Council on Physical Fitness and Sports (1996). What you need to know about the Surgeon General's Report on Physical Activity and Health. *Physical Activity and Fitness Digest,* 2 (6): 1-7.

Ramsden, Susan (1994). Developing programs for the disabled in your YMCA. *Perspective,* 20 (4): 30-31.

Research Alert (1999). 17 (6): 1, 3.

Risch, S., Nowell, N., Pollock, M., et al. (1993). Lumbar strengthening in chronic low back pain patients. *Spine,* 18: 232-238.

Schack, Fred (1991). Effects of exercise on selected physical fitness components of an ambulatory quadriplegic. *Palaestra,* 7 (3) : 18 (6) (Spring).

Schulz, R., and Decker S. (1985, May). Long-term adjustment to physical disability: the role of social support, perceived control, and self-blame. *Journal of Personality and Social Psychology,* 48 (5), 1162-1172.

Singh, N., Clements, K., and Fiatarone, M. (1997). A randomized controlled trial of progressive resistance training in depressed elders. *Journal of Gerontology,* 52A (1): M27-M35.

Spinal Cord Injury: Spinal Cord 101, Basic Anatomy (1999), www.spinalinjury.net.

Starkey, D., Pollock, M., Ishida, Y., et al. (1996). Effect of resistance training volume on strength and muscle thickness. *Medicine and Science in Sports and Exercise,* 28 (10): 1311-1320.

Stewart, K., Mason, M., and Kelemen, M. (1988). Three-year participation in circuit weight training improves muscular strength and self-efficacy in cardiac patients. *Journal of Cardiopulmonary Rehabilitation* 8: 292-296.

Stone, M., Blessing, D., Byrd, R., et al. (1982). Physiological effects of a short term resistive training program on middle-aged untrained men. *National Strength and Conditioning Association Journal,* 4: 16-20.

Sudy, M. (Editor) (1991). *Personal Trainer Manual.* San Diego, California: American Council on Exercise.

Trieschmann, R. (1988). Spinal Cord Injuries: Psychological, Social, and Vocational Rebilitation, 2nd Edition. Demos Publications, New York, New York.

Tufts University Diet and Nutrition Letter (1994). Never too late to build up your muscle. 12: 6-7 (September).

Vander, L., et al. (1986). Acute cardiovascular responses to Nautilus exercise in cardiac patients: Implications for exercise training. *Annals of Sports Medicine* 2: 165-169.

Westcott, W. (1986). Strength training and blood pressure. *American Fitness Quarterly,* 5 (3): 38-39.

Westcott, W. (1987). *Building Strength at the YMCA.* Chicago, Illinois: YMCA of the USA.

Westcott, W. (1991). *Strength Fitness: Physiological Principles and Training Techniques,* 3rd edition, Dubuque, IA: Wm. C. Brown.

Westcott, W. (1992a). The magic of fast fitness: They enjoy it more and do it less. *Perspective,* 18:1, 14-16.

Westcott, W. (1992b). Offer members a weight-loss program that really works. *Perspective,* 18 (5): 27-29.

Westcott, W. (1993). Regular vs. slow Nautilus training. *The Forerunner Nautilus Newsletter,* 1 (6): 1.

Westcott, W. (1994). Exercise speed and strength development. *American Fitness Quarterly,* 3 (3): 20-21.

Westcott, W. (1995a). How to take them from sedentary to active. *IDEA Today,* 13(7): 46-54.

Westcott, W. (1995b). *Strength Fitness: Fourth Edition,* Dubuque, Iowa: Brown and Benchmark.

Westcott, W. (1996a). *Building Strength and Stamina: New Nautilus Training for Total Fitness.* Champaign, IL: Human Kinetics.

Westcott, W. (1996b). Make your method count. *Nautilus Magazine,* 5 (2): 3-5.

Westcott, W. (1997). Strength training 201. *Fitness Management,* 13 (7): 33-35.

Westcott, W. (1999). Small classes effective for adult fitness. *Strength and Conditioning,* 21 (2): 44-48.

Westcott, W., Clegett, E., and Glover, S. (1999). Effects of strength training on young, female figure skaters. Abstract.

Westcott, W., and Faigenbaum, A. (1998). Sensible strength training during youth. *IDEA Health and Fitness Source,* 16(8): 32-39.

Westcott, W. and Guy, J. (1996). A physical evolution: Sedentary adults see marked improvements in as little as two days a week. *IDEA Today,* 14 (9): 58-65.

Westcott, W., and Howes, B. (1983). Blood pressure response during weight training exercise. *National Strength and Conditioning Association Journal* 5: 67-71.

Westcott, W. and La Rosa Loud, R. (1999). Strength, stretch and stamina. *Fitness Management,* 15 (6): 44-45.

Westcott, W. and La Rosa Loud, R. (2000a). Stretching for strength. *Fitness Management,* 16(7): 44-46.

Westcott, W. and La Rosa Loud, R. (2000b). Research on repetition ranges. *Master Trainer,* 10(4): 16-18.

Westcott, W. and O'Grady, S. (1998). Strength training and cardiac rehab. *IDEA Personal Trainer,* 9 (2): 41-46.

Westcott, W., and Pappas, M. (1987). Immediate effects of circuit strength training on blood pressure. *American Fitness Quarterly,* 6 (3): 43-44.

Westcott, W., and Urmston, J. (1995). The Nautilus Strength Training Certification Textbook. Huntersville, NC: Nautilus International.

Westcott, W., Dolan, F., and Cavicchi, T. (1996). Golf and strength training are compatible activities. *Strength and Conditioning,* 18 (4): 54-56.

Westcott, W., La Rosa Loud, R., Clegget, E., and Glover, S. (1999). Effects of regular and slow speed training on muscle strength. *Master Trainer* 9 (4): 14-17.

Westcott, W., Reinl, G., and Califano, D. (2000). Strength training elderly nursing home patients. *Senior Fitness Bulletin* (in press).

Westcott, W., Tolken, J., and Wessner, B. (1995). School-based conditioning programs for physically unfit children. *Strength and Conditioning,* 17: 5-9.

About the Authors

Wayne L. Westcott, Ph.D., is Fitness Research Director at the South Shore YMCA in Quincy, Massachusetts, where he conducts studies on strength training with youth, adults and seniors, as well as special populations. Dr. Westcott has authored more than a dozen books on strength training, and has written hundreds of articles related to resistance exercise and physical fitness. He has also lectured extensively throughout the United States, Canada, and Europe on sensible strength exercise. Dr. Westcott has served as a fitness advisor to the President's Council on Physical Fitness and Sports, the YMCA of the USA, the Governor's Committee on Physical Fitness and Sports, the International Association of Fitness Professionals, the American Council on Exercise, the American Senior Fitness Association, the National Youth Sports Safety Foundation, and the National Strength Professionals Association. He has also served on the editorial board for numerous publications, including *Shape, Fitness, Prevention, Men's Health, Club Industry, American Fitness Quarterly, and Nautilus Magazine.* His contributions to the field of fitness have been widely recognized, as evidenced by the following professional honors: Lifetime Achievement Award from the International Association of Fitness Professionals; Healthy American Fitness Leader Award from the President's Council on Physical Fitness and Sports; Lifetime Achievement Award from the Governor's Committee on Physical Fitness and Sports; Roberts-Gulick Memorial Award from the YMCA Association of Professional Directors; and NOVA 7 Award for Program Excellence from *Fitness Management Magazine.* Dr. Westcott and his wife, Claudia, reside in Abington, Massachusetts.

Susan F. Ramsden is Fitness Administrative Director at the South Shore YMCA in Quincy, Massachusetts, where she is responsible for the logistical aspects of all research programs. Ms. Ramsden designed and developed the Partnership Program, which provides supervised strength exercise for people with various disabilities, as modeled in chapter ten of this book, entitled *Workouts on Wheels.* She has served on the Senior Fitness Subcommittee of the Governor's Committee on Physical Fitness and Sports, and in 1998 received the Outstanding Service Award from this committee. She is publisher/editor of a monthly health and fitness newsletter called *The Motivator,* which features articles by many of the foremost professionals in the fields of health, fitness and nutrition, and also writes and edits other articles and publications. Ms. Ramsden has assisted Dr. Westcott with several books, including a chapter on practical approaches to sensible nutrition for young people. Ms. Ramsden, a fitness enthusiast and regular strength trainer, lives in Brockton, Massachusetts.